VOLUME ONE

Current practice in oncologic nursing

Edited by

BARBARA HOLZ PETERSON, R.N., M.S.N.

Nurse Practitioner, Ambulatory Care,
Veterans Administration Hospital,
Seattle, Washington

CAROLYN JO KELLOGG, R.N., M.S.

Academic Counselor,
University of Washington School of Nursing,
Seattle, Washington

The C. V. Mosby Company

Saint Louis   1976

Library of Congress Cataloging in Publication Data

Main entry under title:

Current practice in oncologic nursing.

    Bibliography: p.
    Includes index.
    1. Cancer nursing. I. Peterson, Barbara Holz,
1941-   II. Kellogg, Carolyn Jo, 1946-
[DNLM: 1. Neoplasms—Nursing. WY156976]
RC266.C87   610.73′6   75-31734
ISBN 0-8016-3791-0

VH/VH/VH 9 8 7 6 5 4 3 2 1

Contributors

JUDITH ATWOOD, R.N., M.N.

Clinical Nurse Specialist, I.C.U./C.C.U., Harborview Medical Center,
Seattle, Washington

PATRICIA BLESSING, B.S.

Madison Public School Hospital Teacher, University of Wisconsin Hospitals,
Madison, Wisconsin

MICHAEL CHOUINARD, M.D.

Assistant Professor, Department of Medicine, Section of Hematology/Oncology,
St. Louis University, St. Louis, Missouri

CONSTANCE MARY CLARK, R.N., M.S.N.

Clinical Nurse Specialist, Neurosurgery and Urology, St. Joseph Mercy Hospital,
Ann Arbor, Michigan

JOSEPHINE KELLY CRAYTOR, R.N., M.S.

Associate Professor of Nursing and Associate Director for Oncology Nursing,
University of Rochester Cancer Center,
Rochester, New York

CAROL L. CROFT, R.N., B.S.N.

Staff Nurse, Tumor Institute, Swedish Hospital Medical Center,
Seattle, Washington

JOYCE ANN HARLEY DOAN, R.N., B.S.N.

Clinical Coordinator, Cancer Lifeline, Inc., Seattle, Washington

MARYLIN JANE DODD, R.N., M.N.

Instructor, University of Washington School of Nursing,
Seattle, Washington

GEORGE J. HILL, II, M.D.

Professor of Surgery, Department of Surgery, Washington University–Barnes Hospital,
St. Louis, Missouri

JEANETTE KOWALSKI, R.N., M.S.N.

Instructor, St. Louis University School of Nursing and Allied Health Professions,
St. Louis, Missouri

CAROLYN A. LIVINGSTON, R.N., M.N.

Instructor, University of Washington School of Nursing,
Seattle, Washington

VICKI ELIZABETH LONG

Senior Nursing Student, University of Washington School of Nursing,
Seattle, Washington

CYNTHIA ALLISON MANTZ, R.N.

Nurse Oncologist, Department of Surgery, Washington University–Barnes Hospital,
St. Louis, Missouri

P. M. MacELVEEN, Ph.D.

Assistant Professor, Department of Psychosocial Nursing,
University of Washington School of Nursing,
Seattle, Washington

JANET ALMETER McNALLY, R.N., M.S.

Nurse Clinician, Research Project, Strong Memorial Hospital,
Rochester, New York

MARGARET LAWLEY MORSE, R.N., M.S.

Clinical Nursing Specialist, Pediatric Hematology-Oncology,
Riley Hospital for Children, Indiana University Medical Center,
Indianapolis, Indiana

PEGGY JUNE NASLUND NELSON, R.N.

Nurse Oncologist, Department of Surgery, Washington University–Barnes Hospital,
St. Louis, Missouri

MAUREEN B. NILAND, R.N., M.S.

Assistant Professor, University of Washington School of Nursing,
Seattle, Washington

ANN ELISABETH PAULEN, R.N., M.S., F.A.A.N.

Clinical Nurse Specialist–Assistant Clinical Professor,
University of Wisconsin Center for Health Sciences,
Madison, Wisconsin

DOLLY K. REINER, R.N., M.N.

Psychotherapist, private practice, New York, New York

ANNIE STOKES SAKAGUCHI, R.N., M.N.

Head Nurse Clinician, Breast Cancer Detection Center,
Virginia Mason Medical Center,
Seattle, Washington

SAUNDRA ELAINE SAUNDERS, R.N., M.S.N., M.S.Ed.

Clinical Nurse Specialist in Gynecology–Clinical Instructor,
University of Wisconsin Center for Health Sciences,
Madison, Wisconsin

ANNETTE R. TEALEY, R.N., M.S.

Clinical Nurse Specialist in Radiotherapy, University of
Wisconsin Center for Health Sciences,
Madison, Wisconsin

KATHLEEN M. THANEY, R.N., M.S.

Nurse Clinician, Radiation Oncology, University of Rochester Cancer Center,
Rochester, New York

MARGIE J. VAN METER, R.N., M.S.

Clinical Nursing Specialist in Neurosurgery, University Hospital,
Ann Arbor, Michigan

ELISE T. WEAR, R.N., M.S.

Clinical Nursing Specialist in Pediatric Hematology-Oncology,
University of Wisconsin Center for Health Sciences,
Madison, Wisconsin

SUSAN LYNN ZIMMERMAN, R.N., M.S.N.

Clinical Nurse Specialist, University Hospital, Seattle, Washington

To our children

Kirstin and Drew

Preface

Recent developments in cancer research have greatly revolutionized the care of the cancer patient, and nurses have been intimately involved in the coordination and delivery of this care. This book was designed with the cancer nursing specialist in mind but is also meant to update others who are involved with patients who have or had cancer as part of their diagnosis. Its purpose is to present the many roles nurses fulfill and the significant contributions they make from the detection clinic to terminal care at home.

In many cases the diagnosis of cancer no longer requires the totally pessimistic attitude often expressed by physicians, nurses, and the society in which we live. "Cures" in cancer are being made, life is being extended, and the disorganized cellular growth is being controlled. New approaches to treatment and an increased emphasis on finding efficient and effective detection methods have aided in this control. Communication with the general public to increase awareness and dispel fears has also contributed greatly.

Five broad categories are covered: (1) professional awareness, (2) screening and early detection, (3) therapy, (4) maximizing the quality of life, and (5) rehabilitation.

The theme throughout is on the nursing process, with pertinent assessment tools preceding the chapters to which they specifically apply. An additional focus is on openness in communication. New approaches to this are presented, such as contracting with the patient for the care desired.

To give a broad perspective the editors have selected contributors from seven states, representing fourteen cancer centers. These authors share valuable experience in dealing with the new approaches and treatments and demonstrate the genuine use of self needed to bring cancer patients to a dignified death. It is hoped that the reader will come away with increased awareness and reduced fear of the complex nursing care required by the patient with cancer. It is one of the most satisfying and challenging areas in which to become involved.

We would like to thank Ken Kellogg for his patience and encouragement and Pat Tilbian, Jennifer Andrys, and Gina Gross for their typing assistance.

Barbara Holz Peterson
Carolyn Jo Kellogg

Contents

Current practice in oncologic nursing

part I

PROFESSIONAL AWARENESS

The first two chapters were chosen for the introductory part of this book because both present the idea of openness. This openness of discussion with the patient of what was until recently a taboo subject is a vital concept. We as editors hope to encourage greater awareness of this concept on the part of health care professionals who work with cancer patients.

The following chapters, written by Dolly Reiner, Maureen Niland, and Judith Atwood, present some new and humanistic approaches in the care of patients who have cancer. Informed consent and contracting with patients for their daily care are challenging concepts for the nurse. Talking with patients about their problems in dealing with a disease that may be terminal has only recently been encouraged. In the past, patients who were dying were pitied. Staff persons complained that they did not know what to say to the dying person or his family. Many patients were not told their diagnosis, although everyone else knew. Death was a taboo subject until Kübler-Ross in the 1960s encouraged a change in this attitude.

Ms. Reiner discusses not only the challenge of telling the patient about his diagnosis but also the pros and cons of telling the patient the risks involved with the various courses of treatment of the disease.

Ms. Niland and Ms. Atwood present the idea of the patient's controlling the day-to-day care he receives by contracting with the staff.

1 The doctrine of informed consent

a therapeutic dilemma for nurses

DOLLY K. REINER

Malignant neoplasms are rated as the second highest cause of death in the United States, but cancer is the disease entity people fear most. So great is the national dread of cancer that many patients, faced with an undiagnosed life-threatening illness, smile with gratitude and relief when informed that cancer is not their problem. The anxieties and fears expressed by the person with a diagnosis of cancer can be readily understood when we realize that the average American is more fearful of cancer than any other disease or event, including nuclear war.[19]

Health care professionals assume that the human organism has little desire to quit life without trying whatever the art of medicine has to offer at his moment of need.[15] The therapies available for curing cancer are known to be inadequate for more than half the medically treated patients. Until cancer treatments become more effective, these patients, including those on research protocols, are provided with the temporary control of eventually failing therapeutic modalities.[16]

Indisputably, therapeutic research is a complex process. The need for scientists to bring research out of the animal laboratory into the clinical research area, employing human subjects, is axiomatic. With the knowledge that most experimental therapies are not major breakthroughs in cancer cure, the medical community has assumed that adequate explanation of the risks and hazards involved is sufficient for the patient, since he has elected to be treated. What might be determined adequate by a health professional is not necessarily deemed adequate by and for the patient.

A unique and emotional component of human experimentation has become an ethical and legal issue for nurse practitioners—the doctrine of informed consent. The central theme in biomedical research should be the value placed on human therapy, which includes the patient's right to know. With the existentialist view that life is meaningless unless one acts, the ethical problems presented by the doctrine of informed consent should be of increasing concern to the entire nursing profession.

ETHICS VERSUS ETIQUETTE

There are many important ethical theories dealing with human goals, motives, and conduct, ranging from selfish hedonism to altruistic social idealism, and from utilitarianism to pragmatism. What is usually called nursing ethics is only nursing etiquette and has scarcely been concerned with ethical theory. It is necessary to make the distinction between the two. Nursing etiquette concerns the patterns of interpersonal relations among professionals, whereas nursing ethics is concerned with patient care and human value. Ethics is not an internal process but an external one, and thus it is a public process.[28]

The ethic taken frequently—albeit unconsciously—by members of the health professions is pragmatism. William James, expanding on Locke, held that experiment and experience promote an ethical behavior, and that whatever works out satisfactorily on trial or experimentation is good. Measured by any ethical theory, even pragmatism, experience still shows that the obligation remains with the members of the health professions to do everything they can on behalf of their patients' welfare.[26]

DOCTRINE OF INFORMED CONSENT

The structural responsibility within the system for the process of informed consent rests with the physician-researcher. Many investigators assume that patient-subjects understand the possible benefits and hazards inherent in the particular research protocol after informed consent has been obtained in compliance with the *Federal Register*.[33] Although the Department of Health, Education, and Welfare's regulation is fulfilled when the patient-subject's written consent is obtained, the patient-subject's human rights are not.

The abstract notion of self-determination, wherein each person has the inalienable right to pursue his own ends in his own way so long as he does not interfere with the rights of others or the community, is implemented by the requirement of consent in research protocols. However, how can a dying patient be said to exercise a free power of choice? The patient-subject, anxious and/or fearful because of a life-threatening disease, can have a very unique perception of experimentation. Can we say that we have recognized his right to make choices concerning his own life, both in quantity and quality? Does the patient-subject understand that he has control over his own being and can withdraw his consent at any time he chooses? It is highly questionable whether the patient-subject understands what he has consented to. Kübler-Ross,[24] in her many interviews with dying patients, reported that these patients have increasing difficulties in communication of all kinds and at all levels. The progression to the final stage of life, death, is fraught with anxieties, fears, and hopes. Most dying patients do not discuss death, but rather their expectation of living.[35]

Traditionally, the process of consent was used to differentiate between medical interventions that were legally permissible and those which would subject a physician to liability for an unauthorized procedure.[22] After World War II, a growing humanitarian ethic resulted in another viewpoint relative to the significance of personal informed consent and its implications for human research.[21] With the revelation of the Nazi atrocities perpetuated in the name of medical science at the

Nuremberg trials, physicians from around the world formalized ethical medical thought in the Nuremberg Code. In 1964 the World Medical Association elaborated yet another code of ethics on human experimentation which came to be known as the Declaration of Helsinki.[27] The Helsinki code is probably the nearest document to a universal ethical code presently in existence. It brought to the fore the patient's right to consent: "Consistent with patient psychology, the doctor should obtain the patient's freely given consent after the patient has been given a full explanation."[27] How freely is the consent given to a clinical researcher by a person who feels threatened by the prognosis of death? And what is meant by a full explanation that is consistent with patient psychology?

The criterion of consent has emerged in one guise or another in most discussions of human experimentation. The concept of consent has been much derided as unrealistic, artificial, fictional, difficult to obtain, and nonexistent.[8,10,31,36] It is important to recognize that the psychologic constraints or compulsions that operate on a seriously ill patient are different from those which affect a person volunteering his services for gain.[9] In the field of clinical research the Declaration of Helsinki distinguishes between research that is combined with professional care and that which is nontherapeutic.[27] A fundamental distinction must be recognized when the aim of the former is essentially therapeutic for the patient, and the primary objective of the latter is purely scientific and without therapeutic value to the person subjected to the research. Experiments on human beings fall into two categories:

1. Experiments for the immediate benefit of the human subject, with the welfare of that subject as an end in mind
2. Experiments in which human subjects serve as a means for collecting information intended for the future benefit of society[11]

The dying cancer patient on a research protocol can be placed in either category. All the factors that make human beings both accessible and necessary to experimentation also compromise the quality of their informed consent.

The courts have recently accepted a person's consent as being valid, evidencing a voluntary product of his free will, only if that consent is based on adequate information about the medical intervention, including its attendant risks.[22] An experiment, defined by Fox[7] as a process of systematically venturing into the unknown, indicates that an investigator cannot describe or predict all the discomforts, risks, and/or dangers to which a subject may be exposed. With the advances made in chemotherapy, a physician exercises a power heretofore unknown in medicine—that of manipulation of the intracellular and extracellular environment of the human organism. We remain ignorant of all possible potentialities of drugs for therapeutic cure or toxic side effects. Is valid and informed consent obtained, then, on the basis of inadequate information? Informed and/or valid consent still lacks legally specific construction and remains an ill-defined concept, although common law sets a high value on consent to physical invasions that threaten the social, biologic, or psychic integrity of the individual.

ANXIETY AND DENIAL: THEIR EFFECT
ON EDUCATED CONSENT

For the patient-subject, cancer therapy is a great emotional gamble. Physician-researchers attempt to do everything possible to ensure the greatest opportunity for a cure or long remission and, at the same time, minimize the pain and disruption of living that even the simplest cancer therapy entails. It is paramount that the patient-subject has a clear understanding of the course of the disease and that there is mutual agreement between the patient and physician on the conduct of therapy. This demands a considerable, if not full, disclosure of the nature and prognosis of the disease and of all known complications and toxicity of treatment.

As stated by Francis,[8] overt anxiety is a common psychologic response among cancer patients after acceptance of the disease. According to Dietz[5] and Weisman,[36] anxiety among all cancer patients results from the fear of prolonged suffering, mutilation, and death. Investigating hospitalized cardiac and cancer patients, Hackett and Weisman[12] found that of 20 cardiac patients, 14 had normal affect, whereas 18 of the 20 cancer patients studied were described as depressed and anxious. Cancer patients complained more often of anxiety, depression, loneliness, and vague fears than did the cardiac patients. In the existential sense, anxiety is a subjective state in which an individual becomes aware of the possibility that his existence can be destroyed, that he can lose himself and his world. The individual is confronted with the issue of fulfilling his potentialities.

More severe anxiety occurs with recrudescence of the disease. The hope for cure is shattered by metastasis and/or recurrence. Depression and denial characterize the stages of progressive disease as the cancer patient realizes treatment has failed.[17] To Verwoerdt,[34] denial suggests a battle against strong anxiety. He accepts anxiety as a normal alarm signal, with repression of, and flight from, anxiety as a common occurrence. Psychologists, researching cognitive processes in learning, are impressed by the effect of anxiety on that process.

Empirical studies have demonstrated that a high anxiety state is detrimental to the learning process of college students. In studies conducted by Sarason, Mandler, Craighill, and others, it was found in all tests that highly anxious subjects could not tolerate any pressure without losing control on complex learning tasks.[14] Hilgarde and Atkinson[14] state that emotional attitudes and anxieties can have a profound effect on learning efficiency. Certainly this premise can be extrapolated to the patient with cancer. Medical mystique is bound up in medical terminology. An assumption we can probably make is that learning medical theory and terminology would be a complex task for the lay person, sick or well.

In a study designed to measure the patient-subject's level of anxiety and his ability to identify his experimental chemotherapy and their known side effects, initial findings revealed that all patients evidenced a degree of high anxiety. Of 10 patients answering a self-administered questionnaire, one knew the drugs being administered. The patient, a 27-year-old woman, had been a victim of Hodgkin's disease for 11 years and had been treated with research chemotherapy more than ten times. This patient evidenced no knowledge of infection and/or hemorrhage due to bone marrow depression as a toxic side effect for any drug she had ever taken. In accordance with the process of informed consent, she should have known. Her knowledge of side effects included loss of scalp hair, increased facial hair growth, nausea and vomiting, and generalized weakness. It is believed by this researcher that if it is difficult for information input to be processed by the patient-subject, the doctrine of informed consent is invalidated.[30]

According to Henderson,[13] most patients invoke the psychologic defense of extreme denial immediately after being informed. If, because of anxiety and/or fear, patient-subjects cannot absorb information during the process of informed consent, and if defense mechanisms are further invoked by the patient-subject after that process, how can we judge the patient-subject to be informed? How can we judge the process of informed consent valid, and the patient-subject educated in regard to his treatment? Even more pertinent, how can we justify informed consent as a one-time process if massive denial is the mechanism used by patient-subjects? This is the profound and significant question, particularly when physicians and nurses alike are noted to support denial with cancer patients. There has been no suggestion, advice or mandate for the repetition of information or human rights once written consent is obtained.

INVOLVEMENT OF THE NURSE PRACTITIONER IN A CANCER RESEARCH CENTER

The ethical guidelines developed by the American Nurses' Association parallel those of other professional codes. The protection of rights of privacy, self-determination, conservation of personal resources, freedom from arbitrary hurt, freedom from intrinsic risk of injury, as well as the rights of minors and incompetent persons, are included in these guidelines.[6] The nurse who states that her involvement with patients in research protocols extends only to her responsibilities for their physical care is doubtlessly an excellent technician. However, involvement requires energy to preserve the patient's psychic integrity as well as his physiologic integrity, since they are intertwined and indivisible within the concept of treatment of man as a unified whole. Cartesian philosophy has no place in nursing. Our concern is with comprehensive care for the total human being. In a clinical research center, the goals of the nurse are not simply to provide comfort. Nurses involved in a research protocol must understand and fulfill their role. Although we cannot reverse the course of cancer, we do have the resources to prevent a dehumanizing process.[17] Patient-subjects are primarily human beings who prefer to live with dignity and respect and not merely exist.[18]

The supportive role of the nurse practitioner is important to both the patient and the physician-researcher. We recognize that a nurse's participation and contribution to total patient care can affect the patient's attitude toward the research protocol, but the influence of a nurse as a possible factor in patient response is rarely alluded to in medical research literature.[6] Perhaps because of our own anxieties and our own dilemma, we have not yet fully assumed our responsibility as patient advocate. Commitment to patient care and safety presents a therapeutic dilemma to the nurse practicing in clinical research centers, particularly when ethical and moral issues are unresolved. Because something becomes possible in medicine, it does not mean that the action is necessarily right or a kindness.[31] As Ingelfinger[20] has stated, the patient with a disease is the most used and useful of all human subjects. For some patients, death may be considered a welcome benefit as compared to prolongation of life without comfort or dignity because of research therapy. It is essential that the basic questions of who is at risk and who is benefited be answered before a decision is made.[25]

Since any cancer patient may improve, deciding when the battle should end requires judgment and wisdom. The decision is for the patient to make, with input of information, but without any form of coercion, from members of the health team. As pointed out by Quint,[29] the dying patient may ask a nurse for help in making the decision to go home to die or to take an experimental drug without assurance that it would be beneficial. This is a terrible dilemma for both the patient and the nurse, and there are no pat answers. Glaser and Strauss[10] reported that nurses tend to go along with research, but if treatment prolongs dying rather than living, they are faced with the frustration of helplessness. If we do not become involved in sensitive communication with all human beings, we have not fully operationalized the concept of comprehensive care. This is particularly true when we subjectively judge and accept the patient-subject's overt behavior as evidence of his valid, informed consent.

OVERT BEHAVIOR AS EVIDENCE OF KNOWLEDGE

Many social researchers, physicians, and nurses believe that patients participating in experimental medicine become extremely sophisticated about drugs and procedures. The patient and his family readily discuss the researcher's shared information. For instance, patient-subjects and family members are involved in and verbalize the numbers of their hematocrit, hemoglobin, mature white cells, leukemic cells, platelets, and any other pertinent blood chemistry report. However, the question is, do they really understand the significance of these numbers? Are they merely concerned with the precarious position they occupy between life and death, or do they relate the numbers to their disease and/or their treatment? Does the reality of bone marrow depression relate to treatment with tumoricidal drugs or the disease entity, cancer? Are the patient-subjects aware of the increased susceptibility to infection and/or hemorrhage because of the administration of many antineoplastic drugs? Septicemia and/or cerebral hemorrhage is the cause of death for a large majority of patients suffering with leukemia who are treated with chemotherapy.[16] Depression of bone marrow by tumoricidal drugs increases insult to an injured human system. Yet, I have never heard a family member describe infection and/or hemorrhage as the cause of death for the patient-subject. For the survivors, the cause of death was cancer.

We must question whether the patient-subject and his family are as sophisticated as health professionals believe. Perhaps the observed behaviors are nothing but a pseudosophistication that we have too readily accepted. Acceptance of this behavior may be a reflection of our own anxieties. The emphasis on informed consent has raised questions about the nature of the dialogue between nurse and patient. The period of advancing disease is the most problematic for the cancer patient and professional staff. According to Abrams,[1] communication is guarded, with silence almost the common language. Everyone is anxious and unnerved knowing that there can be no success in treatment—only avoidance of defeat.

IMPLICATIONS FOR NURSE PRACTITIONERS

The dilemma of human experimentation and its concomitant ethical concerns must be recognized and evaluated by the nurse practitioner, particularly if the patient is to be served. "Nursing personifies humanitarianism, and human research that involves the nurse must be based on this ethic."[6] Consent should never be considered a one-time process. Patient teaching includes repetition of information regarding the research protocol. In clinical research centers, subjects become, in effect, members of the team. For the dying patient-subject, hope for life is not the only possible benefit. Participation in medical research has prestige, particularly in life-threatening circumstances. Being part of the research team, a pioneer in medical frontiers, can give meaning to life and possibly make death appear less absurd. The bond between the research team and the patient can be highly visible, especially the bond between the nurse and the patient.

Withdrawal may represent the end of meaningful allegiances, but ambivalent feelings about the protocol may initiate second thoughts pertaining to continued participation in the research project. The excellent care, personal attention, and attractive surroundings characteristic of clinical research centers may inhibit the ability of a patient to complain and/or withdraw. Some patients may allow the continuation of procedures past what could be considered a reasonable point in order to expiate some sense of guilt.[32] In a life-threatening situation, the dying patient does not make decisions objectively, even in procedures known to have a high failure rate.[16] However, the patient has a right to know all the disadvantages as well as benefits and to make his own decision as to acceptance or rejection of treatment.[23] The nurse can be involved in this decision-making process by helping the patient to know!

If cancer patients use denial as a coping mechanism for their anxiety, we cannot infer that they constructively process the information they receive. It is doubtful that a patient-subject who is in an high anxiety state has the ability to absorb and/or retain the information necessary for a valid consent. When the patient-subject does not have an educated understanding of the investigational drugs and/or procedures to be used on him, then the medical profession has taken away his human rights.

Nurses must be involved past the point of witnessing signatures to a consent form. Humanism and treatment are not separate entities but are inexorably intertwined. Attempting to produce cures in patients with advanced disease is unrealistic, but dying patients continue to be the recipients of research therapy. According to Zubrod,[37] when there is no reasonable expectation for cure, life-threatening or debilitating toxicity should be avoided. When possible, can nurses do less than help avoid that debilitating toxicity? Experimentation involving human subjects should be allowed only when an informed consent is secured, but what is and what is not a mature, valid, informed, and educated consent remains a subtle thing to determine.

REFERENCES

1. Abrams, R. C.: The patient with cancer: his changing patterns of communication, Annals of the New York Academy of Sciences **164:**881-896, Dec., 1969.
2. Barber, B., Lolly, J. J., Makarushka, J. L., and Sullivan, D.: Research on human subjects: problems of social control in medical experimentation, New York, 1973, Russell Sage Foundation.
3. Beecher, H. K.: Medical research and the individual. In Life or death: ethics and options, Seattle, 1968, University of Washington Press.
4. Buckner, C. D.: Supportive care of patients with malignant disease. In Vuksanovic, M. M., editor: Clinical pediatric oncology: research, diagnosis, treatment and prognosis of malignant tumors of childhood, Mount Kisko, N.Y., 1972, Futura Publishing Co., Inc.
5. Dietz, J. H., Jr.: Rehabilitation of the cancer patient, Medical Clinics of North America **53:**3, May, 1969.
6. Ellis, R.: The nurse as investigator and member of the research team, Annals of the New York Academy of Sciences **169:**435-441, Jan. 21, 1970.
7. Fox, R. C.: A sociological perspective on organ transplantation and hemodialysis, Annals of the New York Academy of Sciences **169:**406-428, Jan. 21, 1970.
8. Francis, G. M.: Cancer: the emotional component, American Journal of Nursing **69:**1677-1681, Aug., 1969.
9. Freund, P.: Legal frameworks for human experimentation. In Katz, J., editor: Experimentation with human beings, New York, 1972, Russell Sage Foundation.
10. Glaser, B. G., and Strauss, A. L.: Awareness of dying. In Katz, J., editor: Experimentation with human beings, New York, 1972, Russell Sage Foundation.
11. Guttentag, O. E.: Ethical problems in human experimentation. In Ethical issues in medicine: the role of the physician in today's society, Boston, 1968, Little, Brown & Co.
12. Hackett, T. P., and Weisman, A. D.: Denial as a factor in patients with heart disease and cancer, Annals of the New York Academy of Sciences **164:**802-817, Dec., 1969.
13. Henderson, E. S.: Acute lymphoblastic leukemia. In Holland, J. F., and Frei, E., III, editors: Cancer medicine, Philadelphia, 1973, Lea & Febiger, pp. 1173-1199.
14. Hilgarde, E. R., and Atkinson, R. C.: Introduction to psychology, ed. 4, New York, 1967, Harcourt, Brace & World.
15. Holland, J. F.: Predication of time of death in patients with advanced cancer, Annals of the New York Academy of Sciences **164:**678-686, Dec., 1969.
16. Holland, J. F., and Frei, E., III, editors: Cancer medicine, Philadelphia, 1973, Lea & Febiger, pp. 489-498.
17. Holland, J.: Psychologic aspects of cancer. In Holland, J. F., and Frei, E., III, editors: Cancer medicine, Philadelphia, 1973, Lea & Febiger, pp. 991-1021.
18. Holleb, A. I.: Nurses, neoplasms and nirvana, Proceedings of the National Conference on Cancer Nursing, New York, 1974, American Cancer Society, Inc., pp. 30-32.
19. Ingelfinger, F. J.: The fight about fighting cancer, The New England Journal of Medicine **286:**52, July, 1971.
20. Ingelfinger, F. J.: Informed (but uneducated) consent, The New England Journal of Medicine **287:**465-466, Aug., 1972.
21. James, G.: Clinical research in achieving the right to health, Annals of the New York Academy of Sciences **169:**301-307, Jan., 1970.

22. Katz, J., editor: Experimentation with human beings, New York, 1972, Russell Sage Foundation.

23. Knox, G. M.: Family health: what are your rights as a patient? Better Homes and Gardens, p. 10, April, 1974.

24. Kübler-Ross, E.: On death and dying, New York, 1969, The Macmillan Co.

25. Ladimer, I.: Risk and benefit in human research, Annals of the New York Academy of Sciences **164:**793-801, Dec., 1969.

26. Leake, C. D.: After-dinner address: ethical theories and human experimentation, Annals of the New York Academy of Sciences **169:**388-396, Jan., 1970.

27. New dimensions in legal and ethical concepts for human research, Annals of the New York Academy of Sciences **169:** 590-595, Jan., 1970.

28. Pattison, E. M.: Psychosocial and religious aspects of medical ethics. In Williams, R. H., eidtor: To live and to die: when, why, and how, New York, 1973, Springer Verlag, Inc.

29. Quint, J. C.: The nurse and the dying patient, New York, 1967, The Macmillan Co.

30. Reiner, D. K.: Anxiety as a factor of the cancer patient's informed consent, master's thesis, Seattle, 1975, University of Washington.

31. Saunders, C.: The moment of truth: care of the dying person. In Pearson, Leonard, editor: Death and dying: current issues in the treatment of the dying person, Cleveland, 1969, The Press of Case Western Reserve University, pp. 49-78.

32. Savard, R. J.: Serving investigator, patient and community in research studies, Annals of the New York Academy of Sciences **169:**429-434, Jan., 1970.

33. United States Department of Health, Education, and Welfare: Protection of human subjects, Federal Register **39** (105): Part II, May 30, 1974.

34. Verwoerdt, A.: Communication with the fatally ill, CA **15:**105-111, 1965.

35. Wahl, C. W.: The physician's treatment of the dying patient, Annals of the New York Academy of Sciences **164:**759-772, Dec., 1969.

36. Weisman, A. D.: This question of coping: coping with cancer, New Jersey, 1974, Hoffman-LaRoche, Inc.

37. Zubrod, C. G.: Principals of chemotherapy: introduction, In Holland, J. F., and Frei, E., III, editors: Cancer medicine, Philadelphia, 1973, Lea & Febiger, pp. 601-605.

2 Contracting with Karen
a patient with trophoblastic disease

MAUREEN B. NILAND
JUDITH ATWOOD

It was a sunny day in early April when Karen, her son, and her husband arrived from Nevada. She had come for a 3-month stay in her fight to survive choriocarcinoma. Most of us on the nursing staff had never heard of choriocarcinoma and thus had several early goals to accomplish. These goals included, in addition to getting to know Karen and her family, learning about the disease and planning for her care. Initial knowledge about the disease was provided by her primary physician in a lecture. After that, the primary nurse assigned to coordinate her care (one of the authors) read some of the existing articles, further learned from the primary physician, and wrote up materials to be shared with the rest of the nursing staff. Getting to know Karen and coordinating her care came over a longer period of time. In this chapter we will describe the patient, her pathophysiology and general treatment, and the plan of care, with special emphasis on the use of patient "contracts" as a strategy that played an important role in the care of this patient.

KAREN

Karen was 23 years old when she joined us. She was pale and frightened, and by nature quiet. She tired very easily and at times was short of breath. Karen and her husband seemed to have a close relationship and had been married for 5 years. Both were pleasant to the staff but slightly withdrawn, giving the impression of being very private people. They had married when she finished high school and had always lived in a small town. The trip to the medical center was the first major trip either had ever undertaken. Their income from his blue-collar job had been adequate, but he had had to quit his job when they left Nevada. The previous September they had had their first child, a boy. Two years prior to that, Karen had had a hydatidiform mole, and after passing the mole that June, had no further signs of trophoblastic disease. She became pregnant after waiting the required year and apparently had a normal pregnancy and delivery. In February, when the baby was 5 months old, she entered a local hospital, complaining of shortness of breath with shoulder and chest pain. The diagnosis was pneumonia, but she did not respond to therapy. She developed a pleural effusion, which was tapped but did not yield trophoblastic cells. Serum and urine human chorionic gonadotropin tests were positive. A dilatation and curettage procedure was done, but no signs of trophoblastic disease were present. She was given one course of methotrexate in March without a remission. At that time her family physician decided to refer her to our hospital, since one of the staff physicians was known to have experience in treating this unusual spectrum of diseases.

TROPHOBLASTIC DISEASES

The trophoblastic diseases have been named and classified in several ways. They are divided into those which are gestational neoplasms and arise from the placental tissues, and those which are nongestational neoplasms. This discussion is confined to the gestational neoplasms, which even when present in metastatic form are often curable. Nongestational metastatic trophoblastic disease, which arises from the host tissue itself (usually testicular or ovarian), is a rapid, rampant form of disease that despite therapy usually results in the death of the host within a year.

Gestational trophoblastic diseases include hydatidiform mole, invasive mole (also called chorioadenoma destruens), and choriocarcinoma. The latter two are also called chorioepithelioma, since differentiation is not always possible without tissue diagnosis and the problem is treated with the same drug therapy. Trophoblastic disease is considered metastatic if evidence of extrauterine growth can be found either in the pelvic cavity or elsewhere.

All the diseases are uncommon, the mole being the most frequent and occurring in about one of 1500 to 2500 pregnancies. About 5% of molar pregnancies progress to more advanced forms of the illness, and not all advanced forms of the illness come from a molar pregnancy. All are diagnosed by measuring the hormonal products of these tumors, specifically chorionic gonadotropin in the blood or urine of the patient. Human chorionic gonadotropin (HCG) levels provide a diagnostic measure as well as a reliable means to assess therapy.

Hydatidiform mole is a benign neoplasm consisting of villi that are noninvasive. The lesion is confined to the uterus. With invasive mole, the villi tend to invade the uterine musculature and also vessels. The course is usually benign, and there is no local necrosis. Choriocarcinoma may be confined to the uterine tissues, causing a beefy red, necrotic type of tumor. However, it usually is characterized by rapid proliferation of cells and by early metastatic invasion of other, more distant tissues. These may include many tissues, but early metastatsis usually involves lungs. If untreated, this form of metastatic trophoblastic disease progresses rapidly and is fatal within a year.

The prognosis, with treatment, is related to four factors:
1. Duration of the illness before the onset of appropriate therapy
2. HCG titer levels just before treatment begins
3. Cerebral or liver metastasis (the prognosis is more grave if either is present)
4. Appropriate drug therapy

Patients who begin therapy less than 4 months after the onset of the disease and have a urinary HCG titer of less than 100,000 I.U. has a cure rate as high as 98%.[4] The diagnosis of all forms of trophoblastic disease is established by finding characteristic elevations of the HCG titers in urine and/or plasma. Malignant trophoblastic disease is frequently diagnosed because of the signs and symptoms of the metastasis and a high degree of suspicion as to their origin. For example, in Karen's situation, she had developed a "pneumonia" that did not respond to therapy, a pleural effusion, and various respiratory symptoms, and her chest x-ray examination was abnormal. In the face of her history of a molar pregnancy, HCG levels were tested and found to be elevated, thus confirming the diagnosis.

Treatment for all stages of trophoblastic disease may be accomplished with chemotherapeutic agents. The most common drug used is methotrexate, although some prefer actinomycin D, particularly if the patient has impaired renal function. This treatment may or may not be accompanied by evacuation of the tumor and by hysterectomy. Generally a molar pregnancy will be evacuated by suction curettage, and some physicians will then treat the patient with one of the drugs until the HCG titers are normal. Some physicians use drug therapy only if HCG titers do not return to normal within a reasonable period of time. The controversy over prophylactic therapy of molar pregnancy with chemotherapeutic agents has not been resolved. In any event, meticulous follow-up of the patient is mandatory.

The remaining stages of trophoblastic illness are all treated with chemotherapeutic agents, the dosage and choice of agents being related to the severity of the illness. In the most severe form of the illness (with liver or brain metastasis, over 4 months' duration, and HCG levels of greater than 100,000 I.U./24 hr), triple therapy with several agents is often the initial form of therapy. The incidence of toxicity in such a situation is very high. Moreover, some of the agents may be infused directly into the area of the metastasis, and radiation of the metastasis may be done concurrently. Such patients have a high risk of developing fatal toxic reactions to the therapy and require meticulous nursing and medical care.

Karen fit some of the criteria for advanced metastatic disease on admission but had already been treated with one course of methotrexate and had some of the signs of drug toxicity. After her case had been carefully considered, treatment with high doses of methotrexate was begun for 5 days, followed by a 7-day "rest period" while she recovered from some of the toxic effects of the drug. This regimen was followed throughout her stay, with some variations in the time required for the "rest periods" and substitution of actinomycin D as necessary. She was carefully monitored with a variety of studies, including white blood cell counts, differential counts, platelet counts, liver studies, and renal studies. The progress of the disease was monitored with weekly chest x-ray examinations, selective brain studies, and careful monitoring of her general condition. She developed most of the symptoms of drug toxicity, including dangerous suppression of her bone marrow function, some renal toxicity, and particularly uncomfortable stomatitis and rashes. Her respiratory metastasis continued to develop, and other areas of metastasis began to show up. Despite all this, she remained able to recover sufficiently from each new insult to go on a short, overnight pass throughout her stay. The nurses learned a great deal about observing and intervening in the care of a patient with severe drug toxicity and progressive illness, both of which contributed to there being room for little error in planning care.

Another important decision made early was to focus on curing Karen, not providing mere maintenance care. This decision was made although all of us, including Karen, realized that her prognosis was not optimal. This decision set the tone for the care planning process.

PLANNING FOR CARE

The physiologic problems of choriocarcinoma and its treatment resulted in limited energy as the overall problem for Karen. From Karen's point of view, it was important to be well groomed and vibrant when seeing her husband and child, to get well, and to go home. Because of her limited energy, Karen's goals were at times difficult for her to achieve. Even though she got along well with the staff, her lack of energy made her resistive to care. Therefore it soon became obvious that the plan of care had to focus on ways of helping Karen conserve energy for maintenance of her physical function and personal appearance.

CONTRACTING

One major approach to Karen's care was the use of contracting. A contract is "an agreement between two or more parties."[15] It may be formal or informal, written or verbal. Despite its nature, expectations and goals are made explicit for all persons involved in the contract. As a common frame of reference, it can draw together all the health team members, including the patient and family, for sharing in care and accomplishing goals of therapy. Although some of the elements of contracting are found in other approaches such as behavior modification, contracting differs by having the patient's desires included in the agreements for care.

The first step in drawing up a contract is to reach an agreement between the significant members of the health team (including the patient) who are most directly involved in the care planning process. Then all others involved in the care must be apprised of the agreements. In Karen's situation 4 people were primarily responsible for establishing the contract. One nurse was designated as having responsibility for overall planning of nursing care. This nurse worked with a primary physician and a resident, who assumed responsibility for overall planning of medical care. Together the primary nurse, the two primary physicians, and Karen established the agreements of the contract. Karen's husband had limited contact with the staff and little direct involvement in the contract. He had obtained a local job and, with responsibility for their son, could visit only in the evenings. Visiting time was spent with Karen in private. Therefore, Karen assumed responsibility for communicating plans to her husband.

Ideally everyone will agree with the contract, but realistically this is rarely the case. When there is disagreement, the primary health team members involved in the contract have to assume the responsibility for finding compromises, settling disputes, and altering the contract as appropriate. The patient should not be the negotiator or arbitrator of disputes, but realistic appraisal of the situation may mean that the patient will need to know when major differences in opinion occur, and understand the basis for these differences. Most patients find such an honest approach helpful and are able to handle minor variations from the contract realistically. Karen was able to deal with variations in the contract because she understood why they occurred. When conflict arose or members of the staff did not follow through on the agreements of the contract, the primary nurse was usually the negotiator of disputes. Through the use of contracting, Karen viewed the staff as caring about her as a person and about her needs. The staff viewed contracting as an effective method of helping Karen cope with her problems and felt rewarded by the personalized care.

KAREN'S PROBLEMS

During the 3 months that Karen was under care, the following problems emerged, all of which influenced her energy level:
1. Progress of the disease process
2. Toxicity responses to the treatment
3. Pain and discomfort: chest pain and stomatitis 2°* drug therapy and No. 1
4. Nutritional wasting, nausea and vomiting 2° drug therapy
5. Immobility 2° No. 4
6. Prevention of infection (especially respiratory) 2° Nos. 1 to 5
7. Fear of dying

Problems 1 and 2: Progress of the disease process and toxic responses to treatment

Karen was interested in nothing less than full knowledge of the progress of her disease. She was given as much scientific information as was feasible regarding the course of the disease and how the effects of therapy would lower her energy level. This information decreased her fears, established a trusting relationship, and gave her hopeful yet realistic expectations. She thus became an informed and active participant in her care. Together Karen and the staff designed her care so that she could be physically at her best for grooming herself and for visiting with her husband.

Karen's long-term goal was to improve and to go out on periodic passes until she was well enough to go home. The agreement with Karen was that she could go home on pass if the following criteria were present:
1. While blood count, 3000
2. Platelets, 100,000
3. No infection present
4. Able to perform her own "activities of daily living"
5. Self-management of pain

---

*2° = due to.

To monitor her progress, Karen kept her own records of the results of HCG levels in blood and urine. The results of these studies and others, such as chest x-ray examination and other blood work, were shared with Karen by the primary people involved in the contract. When progress was discussed it was presented with hope for recovery and related to Karen's goals. During her hospitalization Karen received a chest x-ray examination every Friday. Shortly after returning to the unit, the results were shared with Karen. If there was improvement, anyone on staff could tell her the results. If the condition was worse, she was told later in the day by one of the primary physicians. Karen soon realized that who told her, and when, were related to her status. The staff then revised the plan so that on Friday mornings one of the primary physicians made an appointment to see her as early as possible, and this person always told her the results.

On other days the primary physician always planned time to visit privately with her, which provided for discussion of personal concerns on a one-to-one basis rather than in front of the many people on medical rounds. This was important for developing a relationship in which Karen felt free and open. Although she liked other staff and could relate well with them, it put a strain on her to be open with those she knew less well and/or to discuss problems in a large group. When Karen needed information and one of the primary people was not available, discussions were in relation to immediate problems. Long-term problems were discussed with one of the primary people. This type of arrangement was discussed with Karen. The primary nurse told Karen that she would be working closely with the doctors and the other nurses but that communication breakdowns could occur. Karen also was told that there would be times when not all of the people caring for her would be familiar with the agreements of the contract.

When the primary nurse could not share information with Karen, she was told that "this is being discussed, and I will see that you receive the information." Some might say that this was "copping out," but it was believed necessary as a valve for times when facts were unknown or difficult to discuss. If plans had not been discussed and decided on for overall care, then Karen was given limited information. Accurate information from one of the primary people was believed more beneficial for her overall care than giving bits and pieces of information.

One such situation occurred after Karen had been under care for 2½ months: she had a grand mal seizure. When Karen woke up, she asked, "Have I had a seizure?" When told yes, she said, "That means I have it in my brain." Because the seizure indicated to the primary nurse a high likelihood of brain metastasis and a change in Karen's prognosis, this topic needed to be discussed with one of the primary physicians. Unfortunately, neither primary physician was present. Thus one of the junior residents talked with Karen. He gave her five potential reasons for the seizure, all of which could have been possible but were not very likely. He also wrote an order restricting any further discussion of this topic. In many ways this restriction was a breech of contract, because Karen was to be given realistic information. Karen became frightened and frustrated about not "knowing." On the other hand, this situation did provide an opportunity for Karen to discuss the problem with the people with whom she already had established rapport and those best informed regarding her prognosis. It also allowed for group support among the primary people as well as time for the staff to deal with some of their feelings. Initially Karen was quiet and withdrawn, and physically appeared tense. After the primary physician talked with her, there was a visible change in her behavior, and she appeared relaxed—despite the fact that she knew the reality of her prognosis. The point here is not what specific information should be given to the patient but the necessity of jointly deciding the best way to support Karen—by providing accurate information, maintaining a trusting relationship, and being consistent in approach.

To maintain Karen's maximum function and energy on a day-to-day basis, a contract was developed with Karen regarding the level of activity that could be expected in relation to her toxicity pattern. Some areas of the contract were more difficult for Karen that others, especially those relating to discomfort and pain. The agreement was as follows:

Therapy pattern	Feeling	Activity
During therapy	"Okay"	All agreed-on activities
Sixth day	Felt bad	ADL—general hygiene
Seventh day	"Worse" (especially stomatitis)	Only minimum ADL and respiratory therapy
Eighth and ninth days	"Worst"	Light sedation, mouth care, IV, ADL (at least turn, cough and breathe deeply)
Rest periods	"Best"	All agreed-on activities

Karen did well in the areas of activities of daily living (ADL) and usually did well with nutrition. She disliked the respiratory therapy and oral care and would bargain persistently for changes in care. The staff was able to come to satisfactory agreements with Karen.

Problem 3: Pain and discomfort

Through the use of contracting, Karen was afforded much more control over her problem with pain than most patients usually would have in a similar situation. The agreements were that Karen (1) would gradually increase her self-management of medications for pain and (2) could go home on pass if she managed herself on oral medications, provided that she had achieved the criteria set up for problems 1 and 2. The primary nurse shared information with Karen regarding the effects of the medications and how these drugs could affect ADL. She was told the options she could use: meperidine hydrochloride (Demerol), codeine, morphine, propoxyphene hydrochloride (Darvon), etc. She also was given information about the consequences of heavy sedation. After it was determined that Karen understood the effects of the drugs, she started selecting drugs according to the quality and quantity of her pain. As she increased her ability to manage her pain, she increased the control over the selection of the medication. The objectives were for Karen to be comfortable and to maintain maximum functional ability. Inappropriate management, so that she received either too little medication for comfort or too heavy sedation, impaired her physical functioning ability, her personal appearance, and her relationship with her husband. Karen was well motivated for good management. If she managed poorly, she had less control and more difficulty achieving her goals. At no time did Karen abuse the use of drugs. In fact, when she had primary responsibility for managing her pain, she used less morphine than when she was managed by staff.

Some difficulties did arise in contracting with Karen in the management of her pain. The reason was that some staff members were unable to deal with the contract—not that Karen could not follow through on prior agreements. It was important that the staff and Karen not perceive a breach in contract as a reflection of good versus poor care. When incidents arose, the primary nurse discussed them with Karen. The focus was on how well Karen had done in attempting to manage her pain, not on the responses of staff members. Karen still had the primary nurse as a source of information and as a person to maintain the agreements and to help her remain focused on her goals.

One such incident occurred because a nurse did not feel comfortable telling Karen the names of the medications she was receiving. When Karen wanted pain medication and asked, "What is that?" the nurse refused to give Karen the information. Karen had not yet learned to relate the effects of various medications without knowing which drugs she was receiving. She needed this information for managing her pain. The primary nurse first discussed the situation with the other nurses, but there was no resolution of the problem. A plan was developed by Karen and the primary nurse to circumvent future difficulties. The primary nurse showed Karen the pills she was receiving and reviewed the effects of each drug. Although the medications had been explained previously, Karen was still in the process of trying to identify the pills. After this was done, Karen was able to determine what drugs she was receiving regardless of who brought her the medications. If Karen asked for a specific medication, all staff granted her requests, but some staff members felt uncomfortable when Karen stated which medication she needed.

Another incident occurred when Karen was scheduled to go home on pass for an extended time late in the course of her illness. Prior to this time Karen had been home on pass for a few hours or overnight and had managed her pain with two Demerol 50 mg. tablets. There had been a group decision (including Karen) that she could go home on pass for 3 days and that any house officer could write her medication orders the day she was to go on pass. Since her last pass, Karen's need for pain medication had gradually increased. The contract with Karen was for her to receive enough pain medication to provide adequately for her pain needs while at home. Karen had been receiving Demerol and morphine, and she had been the primary person responsible for the management of her pain. On the day that Karen was to go home on pass one of the junior residents wrote orders for codeine (4 tablets) and Demerol (2 tablets). If Karen had continued with the same pain pattern used on her last visit home on pass, this amount would have been sufficient only for an overnight stay. The house officer believed that Karen should return to the hospital if this amount of medication was inadequate for her needs.

Karen had been told that there might come a time when she was too sick to go home, and this possibility was discussed in relation to her pain. However, Karen was angry because the group had agreed that she could go home on pass for 3 days. She was also to be given enough pain medication to control her pain. She had managed her pain problem well in the past, and she could not understand what was happening. Karen talked with the primary nurse, and a primary physician was notified. The primary nurse explained the situation and pointed out the fact that the decision had been to send Karen home on pass, even though pain had become an increasing problem. Karen had been told that the health team was not worried about her becoming addicted and agreed that Karen had managed her pain well. The primary nurse questioned whether Karen would continue to trust the staff members if they did not follow through on the agreement. The junior resident was concerned about Karen's ability to manage increased amounts of pain, and the risk of overdose was seen as a possibility.

In this situation it would have been a breach of contract not to give Karen more medication. Since the time of the agreement there had not been a change in her condition. After the situation was discussed with the primary physician, he decided to send Karen home with additional Demerol, which she was to keep at home. The primary physician assumed responsibility for the additional medication. The discussion centered on what Karen needed for her pain, and not on the decision of the house officer. Staff rights are as important as patient rights; therefore no staff member should be cajoled into treating a patient other than as one feels, in good conscience, is appropriate. On the other hand, it is important to maintain the agreement of the contract to continue a trusting relationship and continuity of care. By reaffirming the agreement, the risks were decreased. At first appearance it seems to be more of a risk to send Karen home with large amounts of medication than with small amounts. However, because the staff followed through on the agreement with Karen, she would trust the staff and most likely not want to decrease the staff's trust in her by poor management of her pain. Safety valves also were built into the situation. Karen had been advised as to how to obtain morphine intramuscularly if she needed it. Her husband had decided that he did not want to learn to give injections. Therefore arrangements had been made for a public health nurse to visit the home if Karen needed an injection. If Karen was unable to contact the public health nurse, she could go to an emergency room for an injection or return to the hospital. She was to decide how to manage the situation once she arrived home.

If the contract was broken and she did not receive enough medication, she would have less control and less trust in the staff, would feel less support, and possibly would have been in a poor frame of mind for self-management of pain. Other alternatives for Karen could have been enduring more pain, with the possibility of depression and decreased functioning ability, or seeking out another physician for more medication. These responses of "poor management" of pain could have made her feel guilty or have less confidence and more difficulty managing pain in the future. Which approach would have actually involved the greatest risk: giving or withholding medication? There seemed to be less risk involved in giving additional medication than in withholding treatment.

Problem 4: Nutritional wasting and nausea/vomiting 2° drug therapy and problem 1

Another problem that affected Karen's physical energy level and personal appearance was her nutritional status. This occurred because of the wasting process associated with choriocarcinoma as well as side effects of drug therapy, especially stomatitis. Karen realized that sustaining her nutritional intake was important for helping to prevent wasting. She was well motivated to maintain her weight because of her concern for her personal appearance. However, her discomfort from the gastrointestinal problems of nausea and vomiting and the oral problems of gingivitis and stomatitis made this task difficult. The goal was minimum weight loss through a plan that was acceptable to Karen. She lost a total of 12 pounds during her entire hospitalization. Some difficulty was encountered because Karen never fully agreed with all of the care that staff members believed was necessary. They bargained for the minimum acceptable level rather than the ideal.

Karen was successful in monitoring her nutritional status. She was taught how to count calories and kept a record of the calories she consumed. Three levels of nutritional intake were established: "worst," "medium," and "best." She was supported by staff in her cutbacks of food intake with the agreement that she would supplement her diet with milk shakes. Karen liked milkshakes and would drink 6 to 10 a day when at medium level. On her "worst" days she was sedated in light sleep and fed intravenously. Perphenazine (Trilafon) was also available as necessary for nausea if she wanted to use it in the hospital or at home.

Oral care for stomatitis required the greatest compromise. When the stomatitis was at its worst, Karen usually resisted oral care. Her mouth was so sore that her own secretions caused her discomfort, and water was intolerable. Local anesthetics did not provide relief. The discomfort from the application of the local anesthetic greatly outweighed any relief. Various types of oral care were tried, but her response was poor. The staff accepted the fact that Karen would do no oral care during her "worst" period. This situation was less than desired, but after bargaining, this limited care was decided as the maximum Karen would allow. Karen did manage well in other areas of care during her "worst" periods. She bargained for oral care to be one area in which she would receive what staff believed was minimum care.

Problem 5: Immobility

Immobility was a problem that lent itself with great ease to contracting. The goal was maximum physical function considering all previously stated problems.

Thus how well other problems were managed directly influenced mobility. Karen was taught the hazards of immobility and did understand how immobility related to her other problems and her overall energy level. She chose the activities she would perform in relation to her toxicity pattern. Although she needed encouragement, she was able to follow through on the agreements. When she bargained, the problem was discussed in relation to maintenance of enough energy for going home.

On her "best" days she took complete care of herself. She chose to take a tub bath, wash the tub after use, shampoo her hair, etc. Making her bed was a shared activity with the nurse. Except during her "worst" days, Karen chose to dress herself daily because she felt more energetic and well groomed when she was dressed. She agreed to nap daily to keep up her energy. On her "bad" days activities were adjusted accordingly, but she still took her own bath and carried out essentials of daily living. This plan was successful both from Karen's and the staff's point of view.

Problem 6: Prevention of infection

Karen's stomatitis influenced her nutritional problem and was a potential source of infection as well. Since a compromise had been made in the care of her stomatitis, the potential problem of respiratory infection and protection from any sources of infection became the major emphasis of care. Negotiating care to prevent infection was difficult. One reason may have been that prevention was a staff goal, and Karen never really internalized it as a problem. Furthermore, some of the measures to prevent infection caused her discomfort. Since Karen was on a research unit, this problem was handled somewhat differently from the way it might have been handled in the usual situation. The staff's goal was to prevent infection that could occur secondary to decreased immobility, decreased immunity, poor nutritional status, the use of drugs, and decreased respiratory function.

The main approaches were as follows:
1. Isolation from other floors in the hospital
2. No contact with infectious people
3. Encouragement of social contact with noninfectious people
4. Intermittent positive-pressure breathing, 15 breaths every 2 hours, or carbon dioxide rebreather, if no infection present
5. Mouth care

To decrease social isolation and yet strive for prevention of infection, several measures were employed. Physicians were to see her first before other patients or change into scrub clothes. The same nurse cared for her throughout an entire shift. She was placed on the unit away from any infected patients. Despite the restrictions, Karen was encouraged to socialize with other patients on the unit who were "noninfectious," and her husband visited regularly. Karen planned a going-away party for one of her favorite residents. Even though she had very limited direct participation in the planning of the party, she perceived that she had planned the party, and she presented the resident with a cake. This was a boost to her morale, and she felt good about being able to do something for someone else.

For respiratory therapy, the agreement was that if she had adequate chest expansion, she could decrease the time and number of breaths on the Bird respirator for intermittent positive-pressure breathing. When she was at her "worst" and refused to use the Bird respirator, she could use the carbon dioxide rebreather if no infection was present. The primary nurse explained lung physiology and the purpose of the therapy and gave Karen cards for the times of respiratory therapy. This approach was helpful, but she still required much reminding to follow through. It is interesting to note that she never forgot to take her birth control pills, but she usually forgot to do the inhalation therapy. She did perform the tasks requested for respiratory therapy, but she had to compromise in this area. The compromise was between patient comfort and staff's desire to prevent infection. Fortunately, Karen never developed any significant infections, at least none requiring antibiotic therapy. As it turned out, both staff and Karen had to compromise on care in relation to overall goals: Karen compromised in the area of respiratory care, and the staff compromised on care for stomatitis.

Problem 7: Fear of dying

The last problem for Karen, or perhaps one should say the first problem, was fear of death. At the time of admission and throughout her course, the overall care had been directed toward cure rather than maintenance. This was considered a realistic goal for Karen until she started showing signs of poor prognosis: HCG levels remained resistant, and signs of progressive metastasis were present. When she had a seizure, the staff began to realize that cure was not realistic. Karen also understood the poor prognosis, although she did not revise her goals until returning from home on pass a little more than 24 hours before her death. She returned from home because of increased tachypnea. Karen was depressed and said, "I'm ready to give up, and I can't take it any more emotionally."

One of the elements of contracting is an honest and open relationship. Karen had a need to talk about her death, but the primary nurse found it difficult to talk openly. She expressed her feelings and suggested that the best support she could provide for Karen was to bring additional help. Since neither primary physician was immediately available, a psychiatric consultation was suggested to Karen. The primary nurse explained that a psychiatrist is a person especially skilled at listening and that this person could help her deal explicitly with her death. The contract with Karen at this point was to ensure that she have a means of discussing her feelings openly and to help her cope with her death. Karen's husband was not an alternative support person because he was unable to discuss death with Karen. He had had much difficulty in dealing with Karen's downward course, since she always had been the stabilizing force in the family. Thus the agreement with Karen was for a psychiatrist to come and talk with her; the primary nurse would be available if this approach was not helpful. Karen was able to openly discuss her feelings about dying with the psychiatrist. Since this was also a time of crisis for all of the nursing staff, the psychiatrist provided support for the staff.

Karen died during the middle of the night 96 days after admission and less than 24 hours after talking with the psychiatrist. On autopsy, her lungs were full of tumor. The lower two thirds of the left lung was completely full of tumor, and the upper one third had tumor nodules. The right lung had a great deal of tumor occupying its space. Moreover, metastasis were present throughout her body, including her brain, liver, gastrointestinal tract, spleen, pericardial sac, and other areas. Looking back at the course of Karen's illness, one can say she maintained her dignity and worth as a person and lived beyond what could have been expected.

Contracting offered a means of helping Karen function as a person. She had information available to give her a realistic appraisal of her prognosis; people whom she trusted and knew would support her; control through an active role in determining her care; and probably a decrease in her fear of the unknown, made possible by open and honest relationships. All the aforementioned points are important elements of the contract approach. Above all is sharing—sharing information, sharing risk, sharing joy and sorrow.

SUMMARY

In applying the contract approach to other patients with trophoblastic disease and/or other long-term illnesses, we have found the contract a valuable tool for providing and evaluating care. This approach grew out of a need to find more effective ways of providing care for patients with long-term illnesses. Contracting is one method of keeping continuity in care of the patient between all members of the health care team, for making the medical and nursing care plans mesh, and, most important, for ensuring that the patient has active participation in planning care. This latter point is critical, since the patient is provided with an explicit mechanism for expressing needs and making priorities known.

Maluccio and Marlow[11] point out that "explicitness is the quality of being specific, clear and open." When the agreements of the contract are explicit, the patient has more control and independence. Implicit in this statement is the belief that a patient who has more control can achieve maximum functioning potential as a person. "Caring" encourages independence and personal development; it does not become protective, making another individual dependent. Sharing in contractual agreements is more difficult but more rewarding in actually *helping* patients to meet their needs.

REFERENCES

1. Alrarez, A., and Fortuny, A.: Inclusion bodies in cells from a hydatidiform mole, Acta Cytologica **17:**177-178, 1973.
2. Goldstein, D. P.: Prevention of gestational trophoblastic disease by use of actinomycin D in molar pregnancies, Obstetrics and Gynecology **43:**475-479, April, 1974.
3. Goodman, L. S., and Gilman, A.: The pharmacological basis of therapeutics, ed. 4, London, 1970, The Macmillan Co.
4. Hammond, C. B., and others: Treatment of metastatic trophoblastic disease: good and poor prognosis, American Journal of Obstetrics and Gynecology **115:**451-457, Feb., 1973.

5. Hertz, R.: Quantitative monitoring of chemotherapy of endocrine tumors by hormone assay, Journal of the American Medical Association **222:**1163, Nov., 1972.
6. Ishijuka, N., and others: Gonadotropin and steroid hormone excretion in trophoblastic neoplasia, Obstetrics and Gynecology **42:**1-11, July, 1973.
7. Jequier, A. M., and Winterton, W. R.: Diagnostic problems of trophoblastic disease in women aged 50 or more, Obstetrics and Gynecology **42:**378-387, Sept., 1973.
8. Kittredge, R. D.: Choriocarcinoma: aspects of the clinical pathology, American Journal of Roentgenology, Radium Therapy and Nuclear Medicine **117:**637-642, March, 1973.
9. Levis, J. L.: Chemotherapy of gestational choriocarcinoma, Cancer **30:**1517-1521, Dec., 1972.
10. Li, M. C.: Chemotherapeutic and immunological aspects of choriocarcinoma, Journal of the American Medical Association **222:**1163-1164, Nov., 1972.
11. Maluccio, A. N., and Marlow, W. D.: The case for the contract, Social Work **19:**28-35, Jan., 1974.
12. Mihatsch, M. J., and others: Primary choriocarcinoma of the kidney in a 48-year-old woman, Journal of Urology **108:**537-539, Oct., 1972.
13. Pastorfide, G. B., and Goldstein, D. P.: Pregnancy after hydatidiform mole, Obstetrics and Gynecology **42:**67-70, July, 1973.
14. Physician's Desk Reference, Oradell, N. J., 1975, Medical Economics Co.
15. The American Heritage Dictionary of the English Language, Boston, 1969, Houghton Mifflin Co.

part II

EARLY SCREENING AND DETECTION

The purpose of this part is to familiarize the cancer nurse specialist with work being done in two areas of cancer screening.

Ideally, this part should also include chapters on protection and prevention as well as early screening and detection. Again and again, researchers in the cancer field state that prevention *and* early detection are the key elements to reducing the incidence of malignancy. Nurses are in a potentially prime position to alert and educate the public in practical ways to reduce exposure to the multiple carcinogens in our complex society. In addition, we could be the role models for developing and practicing, in our professional and private roles, a cancer consciousness. Much is known about those who have an increased risk in the development of cancer, and we are still struggling to find efficient and inexpensive ways to reach that threatened group.

The two chapters that follow, the first on the national breast screening project and the second on early detection of gastrointestinal cancer, present methods aimed at discovering malignant changes soon enough to enable the treatment to be effective. The breast screening being carried out in twenty-seven national centers has indeed made an impact and *is* discovering lesions early. However, no such optimism can be expressed concerning gastrointestinal tumors. They are still discovered much too late, and some possible reasons are discussed in Chapter 4.

Hopefully, this brief exposure will stimulate the development of an increased sensitivity to prevention and detection of changes in our own bodies as well as to practical ways of monitoring changes in the population groups at increased risk.

ASSESSMENT FORM: BREAST CANCER DETECTION

Reproduction status
Age
Marital status
Age at menarche
Age at first pregnancy
Number of children
Previous history of breast cancer in family
Practices self-examination of breast monthly
Knowledge, beliefs, fears of breast disease
History of fibrocystic disease
History of other cancer
Onset of menopause
Hysterectomy or bilateral oophorectomy
Previous diagnosis of breast cancer
Previous breast complaints, surgeries
Hormonal therapy

Breast status
Symmetry of both breasts
    Indentation
    Puckering, dimpling
    Shrinking or edema of one breast
Lumps: location, size, consistency, shape, mobility, adherence
Skin: redness, dilation of subcutaneous veins, edema
Nipples: deviation in point of nipples, flattening, broadening, retraction,
    discharge, unilateral eczema

Lymph node status
Supraclavicular
Infraclavicular
Axillary

3 Breast cancer

early detection and diagnosis

ANNIE STOKES SAKAGUCHI

Cancer of the breast continues to challenge not only persons in the medical profession but also those of us in the nursing profession. Advances in breast cancer therapy have not significantly altered the statistics of morbidity and mortality of this disease.

Breast cancer is the major cause of cancer death among women in the United States. In 1974, an estimated 89,000 new cases were diagnosed, and 32,500 women died from the disease in this country.[21]

Breast cancer is potentially curable if diagnosed early and treated promptly. Early detection of breast cancer before it has metastasized increases a patient's chance for long-term survival and cure. Patients who have negative axillary lymph nodes at the time of diagnosis have a 5-year survival rate of 75%, and 65% of these patients live 10 years or longer. However, patients with axillary involvement have a 5-year survival rate of 50% and only 25% are alive after 10 years. In 1974 about 45% of newly diagnosed breast cancer cases in the United States had negative axillary lymph nodes at the time of diagnosis.[2] The challenge lies in improving this rate with a corresponding increase in survival rate. Chances for effective control of breast cancer are largely dependent on early detection and diagnosis until researchers find the answers for primary prevention.

NORMAL BREAST

Understanding of the normal breast will aid the practitioner in his role in the early detection and diagnosis of breast cancer. A review of embryology and normal anatomy and physiology can be obtained from Haagensen.[7]

BENIGN BREAST CONDITIONS

Any discussion of early detection and diagnosis of breast cancer will include a review of the benign conditions. Clinical manifestations of benign disease may be similar to malignant neoplasms. Second, a history of benign disease is considered a risk factor in the development of breast cancer. Therefore an understanding and knowledge of benign conditions will assist those involved in detection and diagnosis of early breast cancer to differentiate between benign and malignant diseases of the breast.

Table 1. Breast conditions

Benign	Malignant
1. Fibrocystic disease	1. Paget's disease
2. Adenosis	2. Noninfiltrating papillary carcinoma
3. Papillomatosis	3. Infiltrating papillary carcinoma
4. Fibroadenoma	4. Intracystic carcinoma
5. Solitary intraductal papilloma	5. Colloid or mucinous carcinoma
6. Secretory disease	6. Medullary carcinoma
7. Hematoma	7. In situ lobular carcinoma
8. Mastitis	8. Infiltrating lobular carcinoma
9. Thrombophlebitis (Mondor's disease)	9. Tubular carcinoma
10. Tietze's syndrome	10. Adenoid cystic carcinoma
	11. Inflammatory carcinoma
	12. Sweat gland or sudoriferous carcinoma
	13. Cystosarcoma phylloides
	14. Angiosarcoma

ETIOLOGY OF BREAST CANCER

The cause or causes of human breast cancer remain speculative. However, with accumulation of experimental, epidemiologic, and clinical information, the prospect of identifying the etiology of human breast cancers is favorable.

A summary of risk factors and etiologic hypotheses will be presented in order to increase the nurse's understanding of the control and prevention of the disease.

Factors in the development of breast cancer

Identification of factors in the development of breast cancer hopefully will assist in identifying the few women who are in the process of developing early breast cancer. Sex is one risk factor. One population that can be excluded from need for screening is men. The chance of a man's developing breast cancer is 1%, whereas the chance of a woman's developing breast cancer is 1 in 17.

One of the earliest known factors in the development of breast cancer is the inverse relationship of risk with parity.[15] The risk of developing breast cancer increases with the increase in age at which women bear their first full-term child. Women with children are less likely to develop breast cancer if their first pregnancy occurred before 20 years of age. Pregnancy after 30 years of age increases the risk of developing breast cancer more than that of the nullipara.

Ovarian activity is another risk factor. There is evidence of ovarian involvement in human breast cancer with the finding of lowered risk after bilateral oophorectomy. Also, women who experienced early menarche have increased risk of developing breast cancer. The later the age of the natural menopause, the greater the risk. The association with age at menarche and early pregnancy indicates the importance of early reproductive years in the etiology of breast cancer.[15]

There exist international variations in risk factors. The incidence of breast cancer is higher in North America and northern Europe. Rates are five to six times higher than in most areas of Asia and Africa. Southern Europe and South America have an intermediate rate. The age incidence pattern also varies geographically. Women living in North America and northern European countries have increasing risk of developing breast cancer throughout their lifetime. For those women living in the lower rate countries, the risk of developing breast cancer increases with age until the middle years; then a plateau is reached after 50 years of age.

Presently there are no conclusive explanations for the geographic variations in incidence. Histologic type of cancer, genetic differences, reproductive experience, temperature variations, and diet have been considered as having possible associations with international variations in breast cancer incidence. Among these factors, dietary habits may offer the best explanation.

Another risk factor is benign breast diseases. Women who have fibrocystic disease have four times the breast cancer rate. The mechanism of association between cystic disease and cancer is unknown.

There is a tendency for some families to have a history of breast cancer. Studies on familial aggregation of breast cancer indicate that female relatives of women with breast cancer have a twofold or threefold increase in risk. This increase in risk appears within paternal relatives as well as on the maternal side.[15] It has also been suggested that different levels of risk occur within various categories of families with history of breast cancer. Anderson[1] reports that relatives of women with bilateral breast cancer have a risk three times greater than the women with relatives with unilateral disease. He also discovered that a high frequency of bilaterality of cancer occurred at all ages with familial tendency to the disease.

A history of breast cancer is another risk factor. From 7% to 10% of women with breast cancer will eventually develop cancer in the opposite breast. The following patients are most prone to develop cancer in the second breast[23]:
1. The patient whose cancer in the first breast is at an early stage
2. The patient with a favorable histologic type of cancer
3. The patient with a family history of breast cancer
4. The patient with multiple primary cancer in the first breast
5. The patient under 50 years of age at the time of her first cancer

An association between breast cancer and an increased risk of malignant neoplasms in other sites exists. It has been shown that when there is cancer of the uterine corpus, the risk of developing breast cancer increases 1.3 to 2. Women with breast cancer are predisposed to developing endometrial cancer. There is some evidence that association between ovarian and breast cancer exists. Breast cancer has also been associated with predisposition to acute myelogenous leukemia and cancer of the colon. In addition, women with cancer of the salivary gland have four or more times the risk of the general population of developing breast cancer.

To summarize, the following women are in the higher-risk group: unmarried, infertile, over 35 years of age, with 1 or 2 children, first pregnancy after age 25 years, menarche before age 12 years, with 30 years or more of menses, with breast cancer in mother or sister, with a history of cystic disease. The following women are in the lower-risk group: married, fertile, under age 35 years, with 3 or more children, first pregnancy before age 25 years, menarche at age 15 or after, with less than 30 years of menses, receiving pelvic irradiation between the ages of 40 and 44 years, and with a hysterectomy, especially combined with bilateral oophorectomy, before the age of 40 years.[21]

Etiologic hypotheses

Research to determine the cause or causes of breast cancer has been extensive. The roles of viruses, adrenal steroids, estrogen, exogenous estrogen, prolactin, progesterone, ionizing radiation, and genetics have been investigated in the search for the etiology of breast cancer.

The objective of a search for etiology of a disease is to effect its control by developing preventive measures and/or by identifying high-risk groups for screening and early treatment. MacMahon and associates[15] identify three of the most promising current lines of investigation.

Interest in the viral etiology of breast cancer developed when particles suspected of being viruses were found in breast tissue and in milk of some breast cancer patients.[16] There is no doubt of the causal role of viruses in many animal cancers; however, the role of the virus in human cancer remains inconclusive. The presence alone of virus particles is not proof of a causal role. The direct method (injecting virus into healthy subjects) of proving the hypothesis lies in indirect methods, through immunologic testing and initiating cancer in test tubes. There has been progress in these areas of research, but further investigation is indicated. At this point in the investigation of the causal role of the virus, the viral hypothesis does not explain any major epidemiologic features of human breast cancer.

Another promising etiologic hypothesis is the relationship of breast cancer risk to patterns of androgen excretion. The interest in the relationship between adrenal steroids and breast cancer stemmed from the efforts to predict patient response to endocrine ablative therapy. Bulbrook and associates,[3,4] in their studies of the use of corticosteroid excretion patterns to predict treatment response, suggested that excretion of low levels of androgen might precede clinical onset of breast cancer. However, the theory of the relationship between breast cancer risk and low excretion of androgen has drawbacks similar to those of the virus hypothesis. Neither explains the epidemiologic features of the disease.

Most promising of the three etiologic hypotheses of human breast cancer is the role of estrogen metabolism in the first year after menarche. The supporting evidence of this hypothesis is the association of risk factors with ovarian activity. It offers explanations for the major epidemiologic features and experimental observations of the disease. However, the hypothesis has yet to be supported by direct evidence. If it is confirmed, extensive work will be required to further understand the determinants of variation in estrogen metabolism and the effect of exogenous estrogens on the natural hormone profile and on breast cancer risk before preventive measures can be established.

NATURAL HISTORY OF BREAST CANCER

Cancer of the breast is not a single disease but a variety of histologic types with various clinical manifestations. The course of the disease may be influenced by various risk factors. Investigations to delineate the natural history of the disease have been in progress for decades. Without this understanding it is impossible to establish a national control program for breast cancer. An understanding of what is known about the clinical evolution of breast cancer will aid the practitioner in the detection and diagnosis of early breast cancer.

Clinical evolution of breast cancer

Breast cancer has only a few early symptoms. Usually the sign precedes the symptoms. The most common single complaint of patients with breast cancer is a lump or a mass in the breast. The second most common complaint is nipple discharge. Infrequently, the first presenting sign or symptom is a large mass in the axilla, a sensation of heaviness of the breast, or a pain due to metastasis to the vertebrae. Usually the lump palpated by the patient with breast cancer is painless.

There are variations in the rate of growth of malignant neoplasms. Some are slow, whereas others are moderate, fast, or rapid. The 5-year survival rate is affected by the rate of growth of the tumors. The slower the growth rate, the better the chance of survival. Even though growth rate and tumor size influence patient prognosis, other factors, such as the biologic characteristic of the tumor and host response, will determine the course of the disease.

Usually breast cancer has the following clinical manifestations, depending on the stage of development. At stage 0, the preclinical, presymptomatic, or occult stage, there are no clinical findings. Diagnosis is made by diagnostic aids such as mammography. In stage 1 a mass has formed. The tumor is usually solitary, unilateral, hard, irregular in shape, and painless. It is usually located in the upper outer quadrant. Nipple retraction or elevation, nipple discharge, and skin dimpling may be observed. Stage 2 is the stage of axillary lymph node involvement. At this point in evolution, a suspicious, mobile, and fairly large and hard axillary node or nodees are palpable. Other signs such as nipple retraction or elevation, nipple discharge, and skin dimpling may be evident. In stage 3, the locally advanced stage, one or more of the following signs are present: palpable supraclavicular nodes, fixation of the tumor to the chest wall, skin edema, redness over more than one third of the breast, edema of the arm, ulceration of the skin, satellite nodules, and parasternal nodes. Distant metastasis is the fourth stage of development. Clinical manifestations will vary with location of metastasis. Carcinoma may spread to the parietal, osseous, or visceral organs.[12]

Clinical evolution of specific types of carcinoma

Histologically speaking, 70% of breast cancers are classified simply as unspecified carcinoma. If connective tissue hyperplasia is dominant, with dense, fibrous tissue, the cancer is further classified as scirrhous carcinoma. This type is the most common form of carcinoma of the breast. The clinical evolution closely follows the characteristic manifestations of breast cancer.[25] In 30% of the carcinomas, the pathologist, by their gross and microscopic appearance, makes a meaningful differentiation of various types of breast cancer. Certain types of breast cancer have deviations in their clinical manifestations. For a list of specific types of malignant breast conditions, refer to Table 1.

SCREENING FOR EARLY BREAST CANCER

Hopes of cure lie in detecting breast cancer early. "To most authorities early carcinoma means one that is confined to ducts or lobules or both and nowhere is infiltrative."[13] When mastectomy is performed while cancer is confined to the breast, the probability of cure is 75% to 85%.[18]

Preclinical cancer is usually an early cancer before it forms a mass. By the time a mass is palpated by a woman and brought to the attention of a surgeon, it may have already spread to the axillary lymph nodes. However, breast examination by a physician of women 35 years of age and older every 6 months identified about 70% of cancers in an early stage and increased the rate of survival.[10]

A screening program such as the one conducted by the Health Insurance Plan of Greater New York has shown the value of physical examination and mammography in decreasing the death rate from breast cancer. The study has a one-third reduction in breast cancer deaths over a 5-year follow-up period as compared with 31,000 women given their usual comprehensive medical care in their medical group. Thirty-three percent of the breast cancers detected were found by mammography alone, and only one of these women died of breast cancer during the 5-year period. Mammography has been shown to detect early breast cancer, and through mammography early detection and diagnosis have become practical realities.

Other existing methods for detection include thermography, mammometry, thermoscopy, and the use of liquid crystals and ultrasound. All have potential for detecting breast cancer but need further investigation of their value in early detection and diagnosis.

Modalities in screening for breast cancer

With estimated 89,000 new cases of breast cancer in 1974, there exists a need for better methods of detection and diagnosis of breast cancer. To evaluate the value of three existing modalities in the early detection and diagnosis of breast cancer, screening centers have been established.

Each breast cancer detection clinic is the result of a cooperative program sponsored by the American Cancer Society and the National Cancer Institute. It is designed to demonstrate to health care professionals and consumers the value of using mammography, thermography, and physical examination in mass screening for early breast cancer. The screening involves twenty-seven breast cancer detection clinics in which up to 270,000 asymptomatic women between the ages of 35 and 75 years will be screened annually with the three modalities. All statistical data will be coordinated nationally from the twenty-seven centers in an effort to define the role of early detection in reducing breast cancer mortality.

Thermography. Thermography is a process of pictorial recording of the natural infrared emission from the surface of the tissues examined and displaying it by various methods. It has been used as a diagnostic tool in a wide spectrum of medical problems. Application of thermography to breast diseases stems from the findings of Lawson,[11] who found that breast cancer was associated with an elevation of temperature of the skin over the cancerous lesion.

Since then various types of instruments have been made available for medical thermography. These electronic scanning instruments, using infrared cameras, function by detecting the nonvisible natural emission and then permanently recording the heat with a visible image by means of electronic circuitry. The average scanning device has a thermal sensitivity range from 0.1° to 0.2° C. The scanning speed runs from 3 minutes to 1/16 second. Recent equipment designs have included color display systems and isotherm contour mapping. However, there is still a need for an instrument that will produce a clear anatomic detail on thermal scans.[8]

The procedure in thermography involves having the patient disrobe to the waist and cool for 10 minutes in an ambient temperature of 70° C. prior to the thermal scan. This allows for a relatively constant thermal background against which temperature symmetry of the breast may be measured. The patient is usually seated, and three exposures are taken—one anterior and two oblique projections. The procedure requires no longer than 15 minutes, including the 10 minutes for cooling.

Thermograms are interpreted for possible changes from the three normal thermographic patterns; avascular, vascular, and mottled. In the absence of disease, the breasts appear symmetric.

An abnormal thermogram is recognized primarily by the qualitative difference in the infrared emission from comparable areas of the two breasts. The concept that the quantitative difference of 1° to 2° C. indicates malignancy has yet to be substantiated.[9] Vascular discrepancy is another abnormal feature. Alternation in size of the veins and changes in the configuration of the venous pattern may indicate breast disease. Edge sign indicates skin retraction. There is an alteration of the regular contour of the breast outline, and the contour appears flattened. Not every instance of breast cancer will demonstrate the edge skin, and retraction may develop secondary to scar tissue formation due to infection or fat necrosis. Therefore the edge sign will indicate an abnormal mammotherm, but it is not always a sign of malignancy.

Diffuse heat is another abnormal feature of a thermogram. There is an extensive zone of increased infrared emission that tends to obliterate the linear vascular pattern. Focal heat, commonly referred to as a "hot spot," includes the unilateral periareolar heat, another abnormal finding.

The presence of one or more of these abnormal features is nonspecific and does not distinguish between benign and malignant neoplasms. Mere recording of unusual heat emission on a thermogram does not always mean a cancer of the breast. However, the presence of abnormal heat emission has been valuable in determining the presence of underlying malignant neoplasms that in a small percentage of cases cannot be visualized by mammography or palpated on clinical examination.[19] Even though thermography does not detect every malignant lesion, using it in conjunction with physical examination and mammography in evaluation of symptomatic women improves its diagnostic accuracy.[9] However, the value of thermography as an isolated technique in detection of breast cancer is questionable.

Mammography. Mammography is a radiographic examination of the breast. It is a well-established diagnostic tool and has been in use since 1930. Recent reawakening of interest in the examination is due to the work of Egan,[5] Strax and colleagues,[22] and Wolfe,[25] who have demonstrated the accuracy of mammography as well as its potential for use in mass screening.

Indications for mammography include a dominant mass or masses in one or both breasts, a strong family history of breast cancer, a history of breast cancer, known benign breast diseases, large, fatty breasts, and nipple discharge. Usually in women under the ages of 30 to 35 years, the mammograms are unproductive. Density of the younger breasts decreases the contrast and details on the mammograms, making interpretation difficult. The diagnostic accuracy of mammography of all age groups is 85%. In women 50 years of age and over, the accuracy rate is 90%.[20]

The most widely used mammographic technique in the United States has been the classic Egan technique. This technique consists of low kilovolt–high milliampere radiographic exposure with a variable target-film distance and precise coning. Use of fine-grain industrial film provides maximum detail. All films are manually processed. Each examination includes at least six exposures—two planes of each breast plus one plane of each axilla. Since the Egan technique presents some difficulties when applied to screening, variations in technical factors have been developed.

One factor is the radiographic unit. Seventy-millimeter mammography is one type of unit now used in clinical trials. It uses an Odelca camera with a special high-definition screen and takes a photofluorogram of the breast. The apparatus is easily transportable and adaptable to mobile screening. The radiographic unit, which is similar to the dental type of unit, uses ordinary house current and employs 70 mm. photographic film. Films are processed in an automatic processor. Reliability of these units in terms of image quality and operational dependability is under investigation.[22]

Radiographic units designed specifically for mammography have also recently become available. Such units as the senograph have been developed for improving mammography. The main part of the device is a special water-cooled tube with either a molybdenum or tungsteen anode and a beryllium window. The tube produces radiation that falls within the wavelengths most suitable for the breast. Results are more easily interpreted due to the excellent contrast and detail. The actual procedure for taking x-ray films with this upright unit is relatively quick and simple. The patient is seated on a stool, and the breast is properly position and then gently compressed to eliminate motion. Two views, cephalocaudid projection and lateromedial projection, are taken of each breast. With this type of unit, fewer exposures are indicated, and positioning the patient is easier and quicker.[22]

Processing is an other integral part of mammography. Image quality and the speed of production are important factors to consider in determining the capabilities of mammography in screening. Xeroradiography has been promising in improving the technical factors in mammography.

Xeroradiography is the process of making x-ray images on a selenium plate rather than on a photographic film. The selenium, photoconductor, coated aluminum plate is encased in a wooden frame. After being placed in the conditioner, the electrostatically charged plate is then used as one would use an x-ray film, positioning it under the breast and exposing it to x-rays. The charged pattern remaining on the plate after exposure depicts the varying densities of the breast, depending on the amount of radiation absorbed. The image is permanently transferred to a paper or plastic by placing the plate in a developer, which brings the plate in close contact with a negatively charged blue plastic powder. The powder (toner) is attracted to the plate in densities proportional to the residual charge pattern. The selenium plate is reused after cleaning and relaxing the atoms by heat for 45 seconds.

There are several advantages to xeroradiography compared to the conventional film mammography. First, all densities of the breast are recorded in great detail. Images are so clear that abnormal tissue masses as small as 1 to 3 mm. can be spotted by an experienced radiologist in xeromammograms. Another advantage is that demarcations between tissues of varying densities are so sharp that the reader can clearly spot the perimeter of abnormal tissue. Its high resolution results in the depicting of minute details of dense breast tissue that film mammography shows only as a white opacity. It also takes only 90 seconds for an image to develop, eliminating the need for a darkroom and its equipment. The major advantage of xeroradiography is the ease of reading and interpretation.[24]

Actual taking of the x-ray films will vary with the type of radiographic unit used and the method of processing. Xeroradiography can be used with the conventional radiographic unit or with a unit designed specifically for mammography.

Certain characteristics of density, calcification, vascularity, asymmetry, and skin changes can lead to early diagnosis of breast cancer. One of the primary indications of cancer on mammography is a mass. A mass associated with carcinoma can be described as scirrhous (spiculated), nodular (knobby), lobulated, smooth, irregular, or diffuse.

Tumor calcifications is the term used for calcific deposits associated with breast cancer. Forty percent of cancers seen on xeroradiography are identified by calcification. It also may be the only indication of malignancy. Some of the characteristics of calcific deposits associated with malignancy are (1) size—smaller than 2 mm; (2) shape—round, rod-shaped, or lacelike; (3) contour—more often irregular than smooth; (4) number—fifteen to twenty are strong evidence, but at times only two or three may indicate the presence of cancer; (5) within a mass—may be indicative of a specific type of cancer (clusters may appear without identifiable masses); and (6) multiple foci of calcifications—may be evidence of comedocarcinoma.

Ductal patterns are another primary indication of the presence of carcinoma of the breast. Changes in the ductal system and an asymmetric collection of ducts in one breast may indicate breast cancer.

Secondary indications pertain to the effect of cancer on its surroundings. A higher rate of metabolism requires greater blood supply. This requirement is manifested by increased venous vascularity, including an increase in the number of veins present, as well as an increase in the diameter of the veins.

Skin thickening is another sign. It tends to affect the part of the breast where the malignancy is located. Skin retractions are prone to occur with neoplasms that are located superficially. Nipple retraction may be another indication of breast cancer, but only if it is recently manifested, unilateral, and persistent.

Mammography with improved technical factors has become a valuable tool in the detection and diagnosis of breast cancer. However, present capabilities of mammography are far from ideal. If the method is to be applicable for mass screening of the eligible population, further improvement must be made in equipment, processing, image quality, available skills in interpretation, and understanding of acceptable radiation dosage.

Physical examination of the breast. Physical examination is one of the three modalities in the screening for breast cancer. The success in the differential diagnosis depends on careful examination of the breast. An adequate examination of the breast requires systematic, meticulous inspection and palpation of the entire extent of the breast, with the patient placed in several positions.

Physical examination of the breast begins with the medical history, which includes information on menses, familial history of breast cancer, other organ cancer, parity, age of first pregnancy, hormone therapy, and previous breast surgeries and complaints.

Once the medical history is obtained, the examiner proceeds with the physical examination of the breasts. Examination starts with the patient in the sitting position; arms are at the patient's side, and then raised. Breasts are inspected to compare the contour of the two breasts, following it from the anterior axillary fold to the midline on each side. An indentation or a bulge or puckering in the contour often betrays the site of the tumor. Asymmetry in size is fairly common; however, a definitely hard, shrunken breast may be a sign of advanced, slowly growing cancer. An enlarged, edematous breast may be a sign of acute cancer. The skin over the breast is then carefully inspected for evidence of dilatation of subcutaneous veins, redness, and edema. Both benign and malignant tumors rapidly growing in the breast will induce an increase in blood supply to the breast.

Nipples are also inspected for deviation in the direction in which nipples point, flattening, broadening, and retraction. It is not uncommon to observe bilateral or unilateral nipple inversion. An inverted nipple is of no pathologic significance if it has been evident for a long period of time without any changes.

Next, while the patient rests her hands on top of her head, the breasts are palpated simultaneously with the flat of the fingers, starting at the upper outer quadrant and working toward the nipple in a circular motion. The texture and consistency of the breasts are noted, and the examiner palpates for any disturbance in the architecture within the breasts. While the patient is still in the sitting position, have her place her palms together and press firmly. Then have her place the hands on hips and press. The examiner inspects for puckering and dimpling of the skin as well as for retraction of the nipples.

The supraclavicular and infraclavicular regions are then palpated for nodes. Usually a node is not palpable until it becomes large. This maneuver is useful for the detection of advanced regional lymph node involvement.

The last maneuver performed with the patient in the sitting position is the palpation of the axillary region. To thoroughly examine this region, the pectoral muscles need to be relaxed. The examiner supports the patient's arm on one of the examiner's arms. With the other hand, using the tips of the fingers, the examiner gently palpates the axillary region. The number and consistency of the palpable axillary lymph nodes are noted. Clinically involved nodes are generally harder and larger. It is not uncommon to feel soft, palpable axillary nodes up to 5 or 6 cm. in diameter in women who may be involved in occupations that result in small abrasions and cuts on their fingers.

This completes the examination with the patient in the sitting position. The patient is then asked to lie down in the supine position. A small pillow is placed under the shoulder and the breast to be examined. This lifts the breast on the firm surface of the chest wall and evenly distributes the breast tissue. The examiner, standing on same side as the breast to be examined, palpates the breast, gently and systematically. Starting out at the upper outer quadrant of the breast, working clockwise and using a circular motion, the examiner palpates the entire outer portion of the breast. The examiner's hand gradually works inward toward the areola, making a concentric circle. Then, with the fingertips, the examiner checks the nipple for mobility. A tumor may grow under the nipple, adhering to it and causing resistance on examination.

The same maneuvers are repeated with the opposite breast. Any abnormal findings are noted as to location, size, consistency, shape, and mobility against the skin and underlying tissue.

There are various other maneuvers that assist the examiner in diagnosing difficult cases, such as simultaneously examining both breasts while the patient is in the supine position, examining the supine patient while she is lying on one side with the contralateral arm elevated, or having the erect patient bend forward with the arms supported by the examiner. These maneuvers usually are reserved for difficult diagnostic cases.

The physical examination of the breast will vary with the examiner, but any breast examination procedure should include inspection and palpation in both supine and erect positions.

Role of the nurse in early detection and diagnosis of breast cancer

In 1965 Lewison[13] identified the nurse's role in the detection of breast cancer: "It is the duty of all nurses to encourage, foster, and promote public education regarding cancer of all sites, including breast cancer. It is their responsibility to teach and preach early recognition of the signs and symptoms of malignancy so as to enhance the timely use of medically and surgically approved methods in the detection, diagnosis, and treatment of the disease."

Ten years later, the role of the nurse in early detection remains basically unchanged. There is still a need to educate the public on breast cancer. According to a Gallup survey[26] of representative women 18 years of age and other, breast cancer is a major medical concern of American women. Despite their concern, only a few women have regular breast examination by a physician or practice breast self-examination. About 25% of all women have not had breast examination by a physician in the past 5 years, and another 25% have had fewer than five examinations in that time period. Even though 77% of all women have heard of breast self-examination, only 18% regularly practiced monthly examination during the year. Ignorance of the value of monthly examination, fear and anxiety, and lack of knowledge of the proper technique of self-examination were the factors responsible for failure of women to practice breast self-examination

The survey also identified a number of misconceptions women had about breast cancer. The majority of the women grossly over-estimated the incidence of the disease. About 38% of the women felt that over half of the palpable breast lumps were malignant. Only 41% knew that the incidence of breast cancer was higher for women with a family history of breast cancer. Of the women interviewed, 43% believed that the use of oral contraceptives increased the risk of developing breast cancer, and 62% felt that a blow or injury to the breast can cause breast cancer.

Such misconceptions lead to fear about any breast lump. The typical reaction to fear is avoidance, which is the reason that the majority of the women do not practice monthly breast self-examination; 46% of the women felt that practicing monthly breast examination would cause unnecessary worry. This survey identifies the need for public education to clarify misconceptions of women on breast cancer.

Every nurse needs to have a basic understanding of anatomy, normal physiology, natural history of breast cancer, harmless breast conditions, and diagnostic aids in early detection so that she can actively participate in educating the public. Each nurse applies this knowledge not only to herself but to her clients in her area of nursing practice. Any nurse who comes in contact with women in her area of practice is responsible for cancer detection, relevant teaching, and leadership in preventive programs. Specifically, she informs the clients of facilities available for detection and diagnosis, clarifies information about available diagnostic methods, promotes and assists in the education of the public on breast cancer and techniques of breast self-examination, assesses the need for medical attention, and emphasizes the importance of obtaining medical attention as soon as symptoms occur.[17]

In some of the breast cancer detection clinics, nurses are integral members of the health care team in the detection of early curable breast cancer. Their primary responsibilities are to examine the breasts and to teach the value and technique of breast self-examination.

In one particular screening project, the nurse has a variety of roles. Not only is she a practitioner, but an educator, a counselor, and a coordinator. The opportunity exists for her to be a researcher as well.

As a practitioner, the nurse is responsible for the physical examination of the breast. Before each examination, she reviews the medical history with the person being screened. Then the examination of the breast is done systematically and thoroughly. The tactile impressions and recommendations are recorded. With knowledge and experience, the nurse is able to independently diagnose breast diseases. She works closely with the director of the clinic, a radiologist. The final recommendation is made by the director after all three examinations (thermography, mammography, and physical inspection) are evaluated independently.

The nurse in her role as an educator is responsible for educating women in the value of breast self-examination. During the physical examination, the women are briefed on the natural history of breast cancer and the importance of early detection in decreasing the mortality rate. We cannot prevent breast cancer from occurring, but we can prevent women dying from it if we detect cancer early. One valuable tool is breast self-examination, which every woman can learn to do.

Then each participant is instructed, by demonstration in the proper technique of breast self-examination. Each woman learns to palpate her own breasts and becomes familiar with the varying textures and consistency of her breasts. If the individual becomes familiar with her normal breast tissue, she will be able to note changes in her breasts. The emphasis is on knowing the normal condition so that if a change, such as a lump or a thickening, is palpable, she will be able to identify the difference. Each woman is told to do the examination with the idea of becoming familiar with her normal breast tissue, rather than with the idea of looking for something. She is told to practice at least once a month. The best time is the day after the end of the menstrual period, for those women having periods. Postmenopausal women should pick a particular time, such as the first day of each month. For those women on cyclic hormonal therapy, the best time would be the day prior to start of the hormone therapy. The concept of becoming familiar with the normal tissue, rather than searching for a lump, is easier for women to accept.

As an educator, the nurse is also involved in training other nurses, nursing students, medical students, and other paraprofessionals in the proper techniques of physical examination of the breast and of teaching breast self-examination. She participates in seminars, workshops, and in-service education on breast cancer for nurses as well as for the public. She also acts as a consultant to interested groups wishing to establish programs to educate women on breast cancer. In her role as an educator, the nurse instructs individuals as well as promotes and assists in mass public education.

As a counselor, the nurse provides information and support for women with breast problems. Counseling extends not only to participants in the program but to women not eligible for screening. When a woman is not eligible for the program, the nurse assesses the problem and advises as indicated. She emphasizes the importance of obtaining medical attention as soon as possible if indicated and will refer a woman to another facility equipped for detection and diagnosis. Simply listening and answering questions may be all that is needed.

In her role as a researcher, the nurse is one of the participants in a demonstration project. She is a member of a team whose primary objective is to detect early curable breast cancer. For example, she could initiate nursing research into the motivational and behavioral factors that prevent women from practicing breast self-examination. Results from such a study should have implications for existing educational methods.

As the coordinator, the nurse is primarily responsible for maintaining an efficient and comfortable climate for the participants and other members of the staff. She works closely with members of the staff in the scheduling of patients.

The nurse working in a breast screening project has a variety of roles in the detection and diagnosis of breast cancer. Working in a specialized area, she is able to utilize her expertise in various ways.

CONCLUSION

There are opportunities in most areas of nursing practice for nurses to participate in early detection of breast cancer. It is the responsibility of each nurse to examine her own attitudes, fears, and preventive health practices. Every nurse should be an example to other women by practicing breast self-examination. If each nurse actively applies her knowledge of breast cancer to herself and to those receiving her services, she will assist in the effort to control breast cancer and decrease the mortality rate from this disease.

In this era of specialization, not all nurses will inform the public about breast cancer and instruct women on breast self-examination. Therefore, the responsibility falls in the hands of nurses working in clinics, hospitals, and other facilities that deal directly with women clients and specifically with cancer. The nurse specifically working with breast cancer, having expertise in the area, is the resource person for the public, her peers, and other members of the health care team.

REFERENCES

1. Anderson, D. E.: Some characteristics of familial breast cancer, Cancer **28:** 1500-1504, 1971.
2. A report to the profession from the breast cancer task force, Bethesda, Md., Sept. 30, 1974, National Cancer Institute.
3. Bulbrook, R. D., Greenwood, F. C., and Hayward, J. L.: Selection of breast cancer patients for adrenalectomy or hypophysectomy by determination of urinary 17-hydroxycorticosteroids and aetiocholanolone, Lancet **1:**1154-1157, 1960.
4. Bulbrook, R. D., Hayward, J. L., Spicer, C. C., and others: Abnormal excretion of urinary steroids by women with early breast cancer, Lancet **2:**1238-1240, 1962.
5. Egan, R. L.: Role of mammography in the early detection of breast cancer, Cancer **21:**1197-1200, Dec., 1969.
6. Gulesserian, H. P., and Lawton, R. L.: Angiosarcoma of the Breast, Cancer **24:** 1021-1026, Nov., 1969.
7. Haagensen, C. D.: Diseases of the breast, ed. 2, Philadelphia, 1971, W. B. Saunders Co.
8. Holland, J. F., and Frei, E., III, editors: Cancer medicine, Philadelphia, 1973, Lea & Febiger.
9. Isard, H. J., and Ostrum, B. J.: Breast thermography: the mammatherm, Radiologic clinic of North America **12:**167-188, April, 1974.
10. Kampmeier, R. H.: Editorial, Southern Medical Bulletin **59:**6, Feb., 1971.
11. Lawson, R. N.: Implications of surface temperature in diagnosis of breast cancer, Canadian Medical Association Journal **75:**309, Aug., 1956.
12. Leis, H. P., Pilnik, S., and Black, M. M.: Diagnosis of breast cancer, Hospital Medicine **10:**33-65, Nov., 1974.
13. Lewison, E. F.: The nurse's role in the early detection of cancer of the breast, Nursing Forum **4:**82-86, 1965.
14. Lewison, E. F., and others: Treatment of early breast cancer, Southern Medical Bulletin **59:**30-33, Feb., 1971.
15. MacMahon, B., and others: Etiology of human breast cancer: a review, Journal of National Cancer Institute **50:**21-42, 1973.
16. Mason, R. P.: Viruses as a cause of cancer: a report on research, New York, 1969, American Cancer Society, Inc.
17. Mayo, P., and Wilkey, N. L.: Prevention of cancer of the breast and cervix, Nursing Clinics of North America **3:**229-241, June, 1968.
18. Ross, W. L.: Breast cancer: past, present and future, Southern Medical Bulletin **59:**7-8, Feb., 1971.
19. Ryan, James: Thermography in the diagnosis of breast cancer, Australian Radiology **15:**70-78, Feb., 1970.
20. Shirley, Robert L.: Diagnosing breast cancer earlier, Contemporary OB/GYN **3:**33-35, June, 1974.
21. Siverberg, E., and Holleb, A. I.: Cancer statistics, 1974 worldwide epidemiology, Ca **24:**2-21, Jan.-Feb., 1974.
22. Strax, P., and others: Mammography and clinical examination in the mass screening for cancer of the breast, Cancer **20:**2184-2188, Dec., 1967.
23. Urban, J. A., and others: The high-risk group, Southern Medical Bulletin **59:** 13-16, Feb., 1971.
24. Walsh, T. F., editor: A new management focus on high-risk patients: developing a predictive cancer profile, Patient Care **8:**133-150, Jan., 1974.
25. Wolfe, John: Xeroradiography of the breast, Springfield, 1972, Charles C Thomas, Publisher.
26. Women's attitudes regarding breast cancer (summary), Princeton, 1974, The Gallup Organization Inc. Available through The American Cancer Society.

ASSESSMENT FORM: GASTROINTESTINAL CANCER

Name
Age   **Understanding,**
Height   **feelings about**
Weight   **Diagnosis**   **diagnosis, prognosis**

History of gastric ulcers or polyps
Difficulty in swallowing liquids, solids
Condition of teeth and buccal cavity
Abdominal pain
   Location and duration
   Description
   Precipitating factors
   Alleviating factors used, if effective

Digestion of foods
   Nausea
   Vomiting
   "Fullness of abdomen"
   Food intolerances
   Foods normally not included in diet

Bowel habits
   Change in bowel habits
      Constipation
      Diarrhea
   Rectal bleeding, stool guaiacs
   Pain on defecation

Electrolytes
   Na$^+$
   K$^+$
   HCO$_3^-$
   Mg$^+$

Blood chemistry
   Hemoglobin   Blood type
   Hematocrit   SGOT
   White blood cell count, platelets   LDH
   Red blood cell count, bone marrow   Alkaline phosphatase

Endoscopy results
X-ray examination results
Gastric washings

4 Gastrointestinal cancer

MICHAEL CHOUINARD
JEANETTE KOWALSKI

The nurse's role in assessing the patient for carcinoma of the gastrointestinal tract will vary, depending on her position and her expertise in physical diagnosis. The role of the staff nurse in a hospital may be to assess patients already admitted. The nurse practitioner, however, may see the patient initially, and skill in interviewing techniques and in assessment is vital in appropriately referring the patient for additional workup and in planning effective nursing intervention.

Assessment is an ongoing process in nursing, and the emphasis today is on scientific, organized assessment. The nursing profession has devised a variety of assessment tools for use in total assessment of the individual.[4] This chapter, however, will deal only with aspects to include when assessing and giving care to individuals having or suspected of having gastrointestinal cancer; these aspects will be demonstrated by three condensed case studies.

According to statistics, cancer ranks as the second leading cause of death in the United States.[7] The digestive organs are estimated to be the leading site of cancer in deaths due to cancer in 1975. The digestive organ sites listed in decreasing order are large intestine, pancreas, stomach, liver, esophagus, small intestine, and other, unspecified sites.

Despite the gains in therapeutic techniques with other types of neoplasms, there has been no major improvement in the long-term survival of patients with gastrointestinal malignancies for some time.[2] One of the principal reasons for this is the fact that gastrointestinal cancers present early with vague, nonspecific symptoms and are difficult to detect clinically. As a result, by the time the diagnosis is made, the tumor is well advanced and has spread outside the boundaries of the gastrointestinal tract. In many cases the patient's symptoms may be specific enough to point to one particular area of the gastrointestinal tract. However, the symptoms are almost never exact enough to help the clinician differentiate between a benign and a malignant condition. (As an example, consider the similarity in presentation of a gastric ulcer versus carcinoma of the stomach.) In other cases the symptoms are so vague that it is difficult to pinpoint the exact location or even to determine whether the symptoms are indeed produced by the gastrointestinal tract or whether they arise from some other organ within the abdomen. Physical examination is even less helpful in the majority of cases, and a mass is rarely palpated in the abdomen, except perhaps after it has invaded the liver and produced hepatomegaly with tumor nodules.

Fortunately, however, the clinician is aided by a variety of diagnostic techniques that are capable of pinpointing the area of involvement. In the majority of cases the diagnosis is made prior to surgery, but in a few cases it is necessary to resort to laparotomy in order to make the definitive diagnosis. Following are some specific examples of the more common types of gastrointestinal tract malignancies, their mode of presentation, and the diagnostic evaluation the clinician can pursue.

GASTRIC CANCER

Adenocarcinoma is the most common tumor of the stomach, making up 95% of all tumors arising in the stomach.[2] Benign polyps, leiomyomas, and lymphomas are much less common. For unexplained reasons the occurrence of stomach cancer has declined in the United States during the past few decades; its mortality remains high, however, and the dread associated with this disease has not diminished. The incidence is higher in the Japanese and in persons having type A blood, but there are no definite dietary or other etiologic factors that can be incriminated in the development of gastric cancer. It would appear, however, that patients who have benign gastric ulcers, gastric atrophy, or gastric polyps are at slightly increased risk for eventually developing a carcinoma of the stomach. The following case history represents a fairly typical example of the presentation of a gastric carcinoma.

Mr. M., a 39-year-old unmarried man, entered the hospital with symptoms dating back approximately 4 months, at which time he noted fullness after meals. For about 3 months he noted mid-epigastric pain that had become more severe in intensity and was aggravated by eating. For about 2 weeks the pain was extremely severe, did not disappear at any particular time of the day, and radiated to the back. For about a month he complained of difficulty in swallowing, until, at the time of admission, he was unable to ingest solid food and could drink only liquids. In addition, he experienced a 30-pound weight loss. Mr. M. stated that occasionally he had melena, but he denied any nausea or vomiting.

When talking with Mr. M. on admission, the nurse noted his apprehension about his condition. He related that initially he believed he only had a "nervous stomach" and thus had not consulted his physician. Then as the symptoms persisted he became increasingly anxious but was afraid to consult his physician because of his fear of hospitalization and the diagnosis of cancer. However, Mr. M. said that he eventually had no choice and was compelled to seek medical advice.

On physical examination pertinent findings were limited to the abdomen. Mr. M. had tenderness in the mid-epigastric region, and there appeared to be some fullness in that area, but no definite mass was palpated. The liver edge was 3 cm. below the right costal margin, but there were no masses palpable. Stool examination revealed a 4+ guaiac stool. Laboratory studies revealed a hematocrit of 28% and a hemoglobin of 9.2 gm./100 ml. Mild liver function abnormalities were noted, in that the bilirubin was 2.6 mg./100 ml., the SGOT and LDH were slightly elevated, and the alkaline phosphatase was approximately two times normal. A barium swallow and barium meal revealed a constricting lesion at the cardioesophageal junction and a mass present in the upper third of the stomach. Subsequently, Mr. M. underwent gastroscopy, at which time the mass was identified at the cardioesophageal junction, and a biopsy was taken that proved to be adenocarcinoma. Because of the presence of a marked constriction, the gastroscope could not be passed into the stomach. Mr. M. underwent laparotomy, at which time a large tumor mass present in the mid-epigastrium was found to involve the major blood vessels in the area, as well as the pancreas, lymph nodes, and liver. The mass was considered to be unresectable.

On admission, the nurse had identified the following major patient problems: dehydration with ability to swallow only liquids, weakness, anemia, abdominal pain, and anxiety. During hospitalization and up to the time of surgery, Mr. M.'s condition deteriorated despite supportive therapy. Due to his inability to swallow solid food, Mr. M. received intravenous fluids preoperatively, thus making it impossible to maintain adequate nutrition. He also received 3 units of packed cells. While receiving his last unit, Mr. M. developed chills and a temperature of 102° F. The blood was immediately discontinued, urine and blood samples were sent to the laboratory, diphenhydramine (Benadryl) was given intramuscularly, and Mr. M. was closely observed. He had no serious effects from the transfusion reaction, and his surgery was performed 3 days later. Mr. M.'s surgery was exploratory, and he had a great deal of anxiety concerning its outcome. The possibility of a gastrostomy was discussed with him preoperatively.

Postoperatively Mr. M. was maintained on intravenous fluids until gastrostomy feedings were initiated, which consisted initially of 1 ounce of glucose solution every 3 hours. This amount was gradually increased when he did not develop signs of gastric distress.[1,3] When dietary feedings were initiated the dietitian was consulted, and table foods were liquified with a blender. Mr. M. was taught to perform the feedings himself. He had no intolerance to his diet, and his urinary output and bowel functions were adequate. Additional aspects of discharge teaching for him included the importance of oral hygiene and adequate fluid and nutritional intake, as well as adequate urinary output and the absence of bowel constipation or diarrhea. Not only was it difficult for him to accept the need to perform the tube feedings for himself, but he expressed difficulty in adjusting to his diagnosis and the change in his body image. He still seemed to be in the stage of fear when discharged. Mr. M. was a religious man and found great solace in speaking to his minister, who was a close personal friend. Mr. M. was to be visited initially on a daily basis by a visiting nurse for supportive therapy, mainly in management of his feedings. Assistance for performing household duties was provided, since he was still unable to be independent. The social service department of the hospital was also consulted in planning for his financial needs. When discharge teaching was completed, Mr. M. returned home. He was to return on a weekly basis to his physician's office for palliative therapy with 5FU.

Comment. Mr. M.'s case illustrated the more common presenting symptoms in carcinoma of the stomach. In his case the diagnosis was relatively easy to make, but unfortunately he had a very advanced stage of disease, which is very common in this type of cancer. In most cases the diagnosis can be made by radiographic studies, but endoscopy is usually performed to confirm the diagnosis and to obtain tissue. However, the extent of the disease and its spread cannot be determined by these diagnostic procedures alone, and a laparotomy is almost always performed. If the disease appears limited, which is unusual, the treatment of choice would be a total or subtotal gastrectomy. However, in many cases nodal and liver involvement is already present. The 5-year survival rate for these patients is very small, and there is no other treatment, be it radiotherapy or chemotherapy, that has made a significant difference in the outcome.[5] Mr. M.'s care also illustrates a long duration of symptoms before the diagnostic evaluation was undertaken. It is unfortunate that most malignant neoplasms in the stomach are advanced when diagnosis is made and therefore remain highly lethal. If earlier detection could be accomplished, then perhaps the curability rate after gastrectomy could exceed 50%. Such earlier detection and a means by which it may be accomplished is currently under investigation and, as shown by the Japanese investigators, would seem to be well worth the effort.[5]

COLON CANCER

Cancer of the right side of the colon gives manifestations different from those on the left, so that the clinician usually finds it convenient to think of the location of the tumor in terms of these distinctions. These distinctions are not categoric, however, and should be considered guides rather than absolute rules. A tumor of the right colon commonly grows rather large before symptoms bring about its recognition; not rarely, it is first recognized because of spread to the liver or because of unexplained iron-deficiency anemia. Tumors of the cecum and ascending colon rarely lead to obstruction until late in the course of the disease, in contrast to tumors of the descending colon and rectum, which tend to produce obstruction early. Such tumors are also characterized by bright red rectal bleeding and blood coating the stools, in contrast to tumors in the right colon, where melena is more commonly observed. The following two case histories illustrate the modes of presentation of left-sided versus right-sided colonic cancers.

Left-sided cancer of the colon

Mr. A. is a 63-year-old married male who presented with a 3-day history of obstipation, as well as pain and swelling of the abdomen. For 3 months he had noticed gradually increasing constipation associated with occasional blood streaking of his stools. The pain was described as cramplike, and shortly after admission to the hospital, he began to have vomiting that was feculent in character. On physical examination, he was noted to have a moderately distended abdomen that was tympanic. Bowel sounds were noted to come in waves and were very high pitched. No masses could be palpated, and there were no masses felt on rectal examination, nor was stool present in the rectal vault. A nasogastric tube was inserted for decompression. Thereafter plane and upright films of the abdomen revealed intestinal obstruction, probably at the sigmoid area, with multiple fluid levels and loops of dilated bowel. The lesion was described as friable and bled easily after biopsy. The biopsy revealed a moderately well differentiated adenocarcinoma. Barium enema confirmed the presence of a constricting lesion in the sigmoid colon. At the time of surgery the surgeon was able to completely remove the tumor en bloc from the colon, and there appeared grossly at the time to be no spread of tumor to nodes or mesentery. Pathologic examination of the removed nodes did not reveal evidence of tumor.

On admission Mr. A. appeared to be quite anxious and uncomfortable. When the nurse assessed Mr. A., he seemed to be in a great deal of pain, had abdominal distention, and was complaining of nausea. Mrs. A., who had accompanied her husband, notified the nurse that her husband had begun to become more nauseated and had started vomiting. The nurse noted feculent vomiting, which necessitated decompression therapy with a nasogastric tube. The tube was irrigated every 2 hours and whenever necessary with normal saline solution. Mr. A.'s abdominal distention was relieved, and his nausea decreased. Intravenous fluids were started to maintain water and electrolyte balance. When Mr. A. was unable to void, a Foley catheter was inserted and connected to drainage. Because Mr. A. was upset by the odor of the emesis, frequent mouth care was given. Analgesics were given for pain.

In preparation for sigmoidoscopy and barium enema, Mr. A. was given a saline enema that returned light colored, with no formed stool. Preparation in the form of teaching and discussion about the procedure was beneficial, and when the results of the biopsy from the sigmoidoscopy were known, the preoperative teaching was done. Since Mr. A. had never before been hospitalized, he was anxious, in addition to being upset about the diagnosis of cancer. His 60-year-old brother had died of lung cancer a year before. Mr. A.'s wife was very supportive, and when possible she was included in the patient teaching.

Postoperatively Mr. A. was maintained on intravenous fluids for several days until bowel sounds were heard and he was expelling flatus per rectum. Mr. A. was given frequent mouth care to decrease the odor of drainage from his nasogastric tube, and he was given analgesics for pain when necessary. These medications enabled him to turn, cough, and ambulate more comfortably and effectively. At first Mr. A. received ice chips by mouth; clear liquids were tolerated on the third postoperative day. Intravenous fluids were continued until oral intake was adequate. Gradually the diet was increased from full liquids to a soft diet. Mr. A.'s surgical incision was well healed by the time of his discharge. His Foley catheter had been removed, and after a mild bladder infection he was voiding without difficulty. Mr. A. was pleased with the doctor's explanation of the surgery. He was concerned about the diagnosis of cancer but relieved that the doctor had apparently removed the entire tumor and found no metastasis. Mr. A. was discharged from the hospital and stated that he understood the necessity of follow-up, which would include a barium enema and x-ray films, every 6 months.

Comment. Mr. A. presents a more or less classic example of the effects of tumors in the left colon or rectum. Not every patient, however, will wait so long before coming to his physician, and it is important to realize that when a patient complains of any recent change in his bowel habits, further diagnostic studies should be taken.[6] Mr. A. was fortunuate in the fact that since there were no nodes or other spread of the tumor at the time of surgery, he has a relatively favorable prognosis. Mr. A. is also fortunate in that resection could be carried out and anastomosis of the remaining bowel completed so that no colostomy was left in place, unlike tumors of the rectum.

Right-sided cancer of the colon

Mrs. G. was a 71-year-old (childless) widow who was a resident of a nursing home. She had two nieces who came to visit her regularly at the nursing home and who accompanied her to the hospital. On admission Mrs. G. was noted to be slightly demented but was found on routine examination by her physician to be moderately anemic, with a hemoglobin level of 8.4 gm. and a hematocrit reading of 27%. Repeated stool guaiac tests revealed no evidence of blood loss, and the patient had only vague abdominal complaints consisting of a vague, dull pain throughout her abdomen that would usually come on several hours after meals. Further analysis of the anemia revealed that there was indeed an iron deficiency, and a workup of the gastrointestinal tract, including the upper gastrointestinal tract and small bowel, and a barium enema examination were negative. It is important to note that the barium enema was given on two occasions, and on both occasions there was some stool present in the colon, the cecum was never well visualized, nor was there reflux of the barium into the small bowel. She was treated with oral iron and discharged from the hospital, only to present approximately 3 weeks later with a distended abdomen and complaining of cramp-like pain. At that time a flat film of her abdomen revealed a small bowel obstruction, and a mildly positive stool guaiac test was found. No other laboratory abnormalities were noted, and a liver scan did not show focal defects. At laparotomy she was noted to have a large, 4 cm. mass in the right colon, which was resected and subsequently diagnosed as adenocarcinoma. Palpation of the liver revealed one 2 cm. focal deposit, which on biopsy also revealed adenocarcinoma. Resection was carried out and anastomosis performed; the patient was later started on 5FU in the hope of eradicating any residual tumor cells.

On the second admission, the nurse assessed Mrs. G.'s problems as abdominal distension and pain, weakness associated with anemia, mental confusion, and loneliness. Mrs. G. was maintained on supportive therapy. A nasogastric tube was inserted for decompression therapy and irrigated every 2 hours with normal saline solution to maintain patency. Oral hygiene was given frequently, and analgesics were given as needed. Mrs. G. initially became confused and disoriented and required a great deal of supportive nursing. Sensory stimulation helped alleviate some of her mental symptoms. The nursing staff checked on her frequently, and her nieces were able to spend a great deal of time with her. Mrs. G. was started on intravenous therapy, and she also received three units of packed cells preoperatively. Since a bladder routine proved unsuccessful, a Foley catheter was inserted because of incontinence. Mrs. G.'s mental status seemed to improve preoperatively. She was able to understand preoperative therapies discussed with her.

Postoperatively Mrs. G. was disoriented for several days, but then her mental status seemed to gradually improve, and she was able to participate more with the activities of daily living. Mrs. G.'s physical condition progressed slowly. The nasogastric tube was removed when bowel sounds were heard, and she began to expel flatus. She began taking ice chips, and then gradually progressed from clear liquids to a soft diet. Intravenous fluids were discontinued when oral intake was adequate. Mrs. G.'s Foley catheter was removed 10 days postoperatively, and she was able to control her voiding. Her abdominal incision healed uneventfully. Mrs. G. was started on daily physical therapy to improve her mobility status.

Mrs. G., her nieces, the nurses, and the social worker helped in Mrs. G.'s discharge planning; she was transferred to an extended care facility near the nieces' homes. They planned to bring her weekly to the clinic for her chemotherapy. Although Mrs. G.'s condition was discussed with her and her nieces, it was doubtful that Mrs. G. fully understood her diagnosis and prognosis.

Comment. This case represents a relatively common presentation of right-sided colonic lesions. Often such lesions are missed initially because an adequate colon examination was not done. The reason may be that in older patients it is sometimes difficult to thoroughly cleanse the colon. A concerted, diligent effort must be made by all the staff to accomplish this cleansing. As is so often the case, this patient had liver metastasis by the time surgery was done, so that she has a relatively unfavorable prognosis.

REFERENCES

1. Brunner, L., and others: Textbook of medical-surgical nursing, ed. 2, New York, 1970, J. B. Lippincott Co.
2. Holland, J., and Frei, E., III, editors: Cancer medicine, Philadelphia, 1973, Lea & Febiger.
3. Luckmann, J., and Sorensen, K.: Medical-surgical nursing: a psychophysiologic approach, Philadelphia, 1974, W. B. Saunders Co.
4. McCain, F.: Nursing by assessment—not intuition, American Journal of Nursing **65:**82-84, 1965.
5. Rubin, P.: Gastric cancer: current concepts in cancer, Journal of the American Medical Association **228:**1283, 1974.
6. Spiro, H.: Clinical gastroenterology, New York, 1970, The Macmillan Co.
7. 75 cancer facts and figures, American Cancer Society, Inc., 1974.

part III
THERAPY

This part was designed to give a broad overview of current treatment and nursing intervention in selected areas of cancer care. It was written by nurses who work daily with patients, and their practical approach is invaluable. It is evident that these nurses have a sound knowledge of physiology as well as a strong humanitarian philosophy that allows them to be effective in their roles, not the least of which is that of patient advocate.

Chapter 5 discusses the role of the nurse in a cancer clinic, information that is difficult to find in the literature. It includes current research and care of patients receiving immunotherapy, an approach resembling that seen in cancer chemotherapy 10 or 15 years ago.

Chapter 6 allows us to explore the nurse's role in drug research as one nurse has developed it. It is refreshing to see nursing's contribution so well utilized.

The increased responsibilities, in-depth knowledge, and attention to the nursing process are also evident in the five remaining chapters, which present detailed discussions of more specific examples of malignancies. They have been included because of changing therapeutic approaches, as with radiation, Hodgkin's disease, and childhood leukemia, or because of the number of patients seen with brain and lung involvement.

ASSESSMENT FORM: PATIENTS UNDERGOING TREATMENT FOR CANCER

Name

Age   **Diagnosis**

Circulatory status
Veins: scarring, elasticity, sclerosis
RBC count, weight, height
WBC count, platelet count
Signs of abnormal bleeding
Capillary fragility
Injection site: redness, swelling, pain, tissue sloughing

Mental and emotional status
Treatment agents and schedule
Understanding about illness, drug protocol (Chapter 1)
Feelings about death and dying
Control of pain
Cycles of depression with medication
Reaction to repeated sessions of chemotherapy

Side effects of chemotherapeutic agents
Alopecia
Nausea and vomiting
Stomatitis, diarrhea
Electrolyte imbalance
Anorexia
Fatigue and general malaise
Amenorrhea, impotence
Hematuria

Side effects of radiation therapy
Epilation
Loss of taste, mucosal dryness
Sore throat, dysphagia
Nausea and vomiting
Cramping and diarrhea, occasional backache (with placement of radium)
Urinary frequency, burning
Anemia and decrease in WBC

Side effects of immunotherapy
Lymph node enlargement, tenderness
Urticaria, facial edema
Muscle aching, fever malaise
Hypotension, respiratory distress
Flare-up of previous BCG scars
Increase in temperature (to 105° F.)
Dusky skin color
Convulsions

5 Nursing practice in a cancer clinic

CAROL L. CROFT

A nurse's role in an outpatient cancer treatment facility differs from the role of nurses caring for hospitalized cancer patients or for patients in a home setting. The clinic nurse offers supportive care and preventive teaching, much like other nurses involved in cancer care, but is also responsible for special nursing actions, assessment, and teaching pertinent to ambulatory clinic patients receiving chemotherapy, radiation therapy, and immunotherapy. These specific actions, assessments, and teaching are discussed in this chapter. Guidelines for coordination of care between the clinic and the hospital to which the patients may be admitted are presented, and general nursing care responsibilities adapted to cancer patients within a clinic setting are outlined, with emphasis on personalized care.

Our clinic is adjacent to a 420-bed urban private hospital. We maintain a minor surgery where biopsies, lumbar punctures, paracentesis, and thoracocentesis are performed, and where intracavitary radiation sources are inserted. There are seven examination rooms and one ENT room. The radiation treatment area occupies part of the clinic area, and an isotope department is adjacent to the main clinic. The medical staff is comprised of three radiation therapists, two part-time chemotherapists, one immunotherapist, and a rotating group of students and residents from a university medical school and radiation oncology group. The clinic manager is a nurse, and there are four full-time registered nurses giving direct care.

The clinic volume is made up of outpatients and hospitalized patients. Approximately 50 to 60 outpatients a day are seen for chemotherapy, immunotherapy, and radiation follow-up visits. Another 75 to 100 clinic and hospital patients are seen each day for radiation treatment. Hospitalized clinic patients and newly referred hospital patients comprise another 40 to 50 persons seen by the clinic physicians per week.

CARING FOR PATIENTS TREATED WITH CHEMOTHERAPY

Chemotherapy is used to treat certain types of metastatic solid tumors, lymphomas, and leukemia. Selected drugs interfere with tumor cell synthesis or metabolism, inactivating those cells of tumor or normal tissue that are dividing at the time of therapeutic action of the drug or drugs.[10,12-14] Hence, chemotherapy can promote the regression of tumor tissue while at the same time giving rise to pos-

---

I would like to thank Dr. Glenn A. Warner for his assistance in preparing the discussion on immunotherapy and for reviewing the medical rationale offered for the use of radiation therapy.

55

sibly devastating side effects in which normal tissue is damaged. Measures and teaching to help the patient watch for side effects and protect himself from them will be elaborated later.

First, the nurse's role as intravenous therapist with chemotherapeutic agents is discussed. It is the nurse's responsibility to obtain adequate experience with venipuncture technique before attempting any chemotherapy administration. Most chemotherapy patients have frequent venipuncture for blood samples and chemotherapy, which restricts eventually the number of sites available for puncture. Veins that are often used are fragile, and they may be sclerosed by the drugs themselves. Chemotherapy patients' white blood cell and platelet counts are frequently depressed because of the drugs, increasing the risk of bleeding and infection when the skin and the vein wall are punctured. Since these patients' veins are literally their lifeline, the utmost skill and respect are required of the nurse administering chemotherapy.

For most chemotherapy, the size and type of needle should match the desired results.[17] In our clinic a 26-gauge straight needle is generally used; this needle makes the smallest puncture in the skin and the vein wall, lessening the chances of infection and bleeding because of decreased white blood cell and platelet counts. If two or more syringes of medication are to be interchanged with a single intravenous needle, depending on the nurse's skill in maintaining control of the needle, either a straight 26- or 25-gauge scalp vein needle (Butterfly), with its length of flexible tubing attached, can be used. When blood is drawn immediately preceding the administration of either chemotherapy or blood products, a 19- or 21-gauge straight or Butterfly needle can be used.

Second, accurate and appropriate preparation of chemotherapeutic agents is the clinic nurse's responsibility. The chemicals are diluted according to the manufacturer's directions; to the type of administration, with the appropriate diluent for intramuscular, intravenous, or intrathecal use; and to the adjustment necessary for convenient dosage division. Compatible admixtures—for example, 5FU, methotrexate, and vincristine—are noted and are thus mixed in one syringe; a chart of compatible and incompatible admixtures, as well as proper diluents and amounts of diluents for each drug, is placed in front of the work table. Tuberculin syringes are used for drawing up minute doses, for example, of methotrexate. Solutions are prepared for use only when it has been confirmed that the patient will receive those drugs on that occasion; some preparations must be used within a specified time period and are wasted if mixed under the mistaken assumption that the patient is to receive them that day. Other drugs must remain frozen, refrigerated, or protected from light until prepared for administration; therefore, when a patient takes medication home to be administered by the local physician, the patient is instructed in caring for the drug until it is used.

Nursing assessment and teaching with regard to the chemotherapy patient require knowledge of the immediate effects and problems of drug administration, as well as of the delayed side effects. Along with this knowledge, effective communication of monitoring and preventive skills to the patient protects the patient from undue complications of therapy and allows responsible partnership in care rather than permitting the patient to become a passive recipient.

Immediate effects and problems may include extravasation of the drug, pain on injection, and hematoma formation. Immediate teaching needs involve the rather complicated self-administration cycle of oral agents; the mixing, measuring, and home injection of the subcutaneous and intramuscular drugs; and the reporting of interim blood counts to the clinic.

Infiltration is monitored first by frequent aspiration and then by cautious administration. If a drug extravasates, especially those which cause tissue sloughing, administration at that site should be discontinued immediately. The physician will usually ask for an injectable cortisone preparation and will administer it into the soft tissues around the extravasated material. In the case of adriamycin, an antibiotic with cytotoxic properties, and vincristine, an alkaloid derived from *Vinca rosacea,* the patient is usually instructed to apply ice to the site.

Pain along the path of the vein—for example, with nitrogen mustard, an alkylating agent, or imidazole carboxamide (DIC, DTIC), an experimental agent— can be minimized by slow infusion and by adequate dilution. If necessary, the administration of the drug can be halted and the blood merely washed back and forth through the needle to prevent clotting until further injection can proceed without pain. The medication should be diluted sufficiently or administered while a steady intravenous drip of 5% dextrose in water or physiologic saline solution is running. If the patient has a history of pain on injection of each course of chemotherapy, the necessary orders for an intravenous drip should be sought by the nurse for the patient.

With the oral chemotherapeutic agents and the adjuvant oral medications, such as prednisone and hormones, administration is usually on a complicated schedule. It is the nurse's responsibility to see that the patient can demonstrate an understanding of how and when medications will be taken at home. Injectable medications may be taken home if the drugs are to be given more than once a day or if the patient lives out of town. If the patient or a member of the family is to give the drug, the nurse not only teaches the patient how to inject the medication but also makes sure, by return demonstration, that methods of mixing and correctly measuring each dose are understood. Written instructions and a schedule are also made out in cooperation with the patient, taking into account home and work schedules. When the drug is to be administered by the patient's local physician, the nurse includes not only written instructions for mixing and measuring the dose and for administering the drug (for example: "IV with a drip running"; "1 ml./min.") but also the storage instructions and any dangerous immediate reactions or precautions to observe (for example: "vincristine causes tissue sloughing if extravasated," or "bleomycin can produce anaphylactic shock in susceptible persons").

If the patient living out of town is to have interim blood cell counts before the next clinic appointment, the patient is instructed either to obtain the results and report to the clinic by telephone or to inform the local laboratory to notify the clinic of the results.

The psychologic state of the patient during chemotherapy sessions should be assessed. A patient needs tremendous self-discipline and acceptance of the necessity of treatment to keep appointments at the clinic when he knows that nausea and vomiting follow each injection. Some patients on certain protocols say that just when they are beginning to feel good and to want to eat again, it is time for the next session of chemotherapy. For some, just the smell of the alcohol used to prepare the skin before an injection initiates nausea.

Delayed side effects of chemotherapy that may endanger the patient can be shared in as nonthreatening a way as possible, so that the patient can begin to handle the information given and act to initiate protection from complications. Because chemotherapeutic agents act on rapidly dividing cells, the hair follicles, mucous membranes, and bone marrow are the potentially harmed normal tissues after treatment with chemicals. Since many drugs cause alopecia, it is helpful if the nurse prepares the patient in a realistic way about the impending hair loss and gives information about purchasing a wig or hairpiece, as well as encouraging questions about the loss of hair and assessing the emotional ramifications unique to each patient. For women with breast cancer, who have already faced the amputation of one or both breasts, the anticipation of further "castration" of their femininity—loss of hair, eyelashes, and eyebrows because of adriamycin or cyclophosphamide (Cytoxan)—can be as depressing as the diagnosis of cancer itself.

Side effects can be monitored and toxicity prevented if the nurse makes the outpatient aware of what to observe. The patient who is receiving methotrexate, an antimetabolite, should know that this drug can cause ulceration of the gastrointestinal tract and oral mucosa, producing pain, poor intake, and diarrhea. Patients receiving prednisone or other drugs that can produce gastric ulcers are instructed to take the appropriate medications with meals and/or with an antacid. Many drugs decrease platelets, thus delaying the coagulation process; the patient must be alert to injury and must observe for any external bleeding or signs of internal bleeding. The patient whose white blood cell count has been found to be low is instructed to limit contacts to persons with no evidence of colds or other infection. With certain forms of chemotherapy, as well as with certain types of tumors, particularly those involving bone metastasis, the patient's family must be alert for lethargy coupled with thirst and oliguria, the signs of hypercalcemia, so that someone can notify the physician for the patient.

The nurse teaches the patient the idea of anticipatory medication, in which medication for pain, nausea, or constipation is taken before the predicted condition becomes established, to prevent pain, nausea, or constipation from going rapidly out of control. The patient is encouraged to be aware of previous reactions to chemotherapy sessions and, if possible, to take nausea medication before coming into the clinic if nausea usually occurs after an injection. When the nurse outlines for the patient the realistic expectations from the medications—the possible depression, anorexia, nausea and vomiting, or loss of stamina—the patient cannot only begin to handle the implications of the cancer treatment but also let the nurse or physician know about the reaction, so that the particular drugs or dosages can be adjusted for the next session.

CARING FOR PATIENTS TREATED WITH RADIATION

In our clinic's radiation treatment area there is no nurse present unless a patient needs a dressing changed or an injection for pain or nausea given. However, radiation follow-up patients are seen in the main clinic, where each patient can be assessed for untoward skin reactions, weight loss, anemia, or other systemic side effects, and proper treatment, such as dietary counseling, vitamin or hormone supplementation, or nausea medication, is sought by the clinic nurse for the amelioration of these problems.

The nurse learns the expected side effects of radiation treatment of each area treated to be able to communicate to the patient these possible responses, with attendant preventive measures and home care. Depending on the location of the radiation field, the following often occur: epilation, loss of taste, mucosal dryness, sore throat, dysphagia, nausea and vomiting, cramping and diarrhea, and urinary frequency and burning. In addition, anemia and a decreased white blood cell count can occur when a large bony area, such as the pelvis, is treated. By anticipating questions and problems, the nurse teaches the necessary preventive care and precautions, and obtains the appropriate palliative medications for the patient.

Nursing responsibility in the care of patients treated with intracavitary radiation sources encompasses operating room technique, appropriate teaching for the hospital stay and home convalescence, and coordination of the patient's care with the hospital floor to which the patient is returned after source insertion. Intracavitary radiation is used to treat women with cancer of the cervix or endometrium (the sources being either cesium or radium) and to treat persons with tumors in accessible orifices, such as the mouth or bronchus, by means of radium needles. Routines such as the ordering of source materials and the scheduling of preceding examinations (such as cystoscopy) and anesthesia vary with the institution.

With regard to operating room procedures, the instruments as well as the appropriate applicators are suitably sterilized. In the case of pelvic intracavitary insertion, the patient receives the usual perineal preparation and catheter insertion. The preparation period provides a good opportunity for the nurse to establish rapport with the patient, to discuss what the nurse is currently doing with the patient, to describe what the procedure entails, and to prepare the patient realistically for any expected discomfort. If the patient is to be sedated, it is the nurse's role to obtain a baseline blood pressure and pulse, to slowly give the sedative or analgesic intravenously, and to monitor the blood pressure and pulse during the procedure. The patient's response to the amount of discomfort experienced should also be monitored. If the patient is to receive general anesthesia (by a nurse anesthetist), the clinic nurse offers physical care for the unconscious patient, with attention to positioning, safety, the length of time the patient's legs are in stirrups, and the length of time the patient is under anesthesia. When handling the radiation sources, the nurse utilizes speed, distance, and shielding, protecting herself and others in the room from undue radiation exposure.[16]

Anticipating what the patient will need to know about how she will feel and what she must do for the 2 or 3 days in the hospital with the radiation sources in place, the nurse tells her first that she must remain flat to avoid pushing out the sources; however, the patient is encouraged to turn from side to side and to flex her knees to prevent back pain and circulatory stasis problems. She may expect cramping and backache due to the presence of the applicator in the cervical os and of the gauze packing in the vagina. She needs to know that there are medications for pain and nausea, but that if she is not offered these, she needs to ask for the medications at the appropriate times. It is important for her to realize that since she has a catheter in place and a radiation source so near the bladder, she needs to drink approximately 3000 ml of fluid each day, both in the hospital and after returning home, to keep the urine dilute and to wash out any organisms proliferating due to the presence of the catheter.

Coordination of care with the hospital floor where the patient goes after the radiation sources are in place can be accomplished by either a telephone report or a note on the chart regarding any special details about patient reactions or problems encountered during the procedure. The nurse notes the type of source (cesium or radium), so that the floor personnel can protect themselves accordingly; rays emitted by radium penetrate lead shields, whereas cesium rays are more effectively blocked by lead. When calculated, the planned time of source removal should be relayed to the floor, not only to facilitate the planning of care on that day, but also to help the patient plan transportation home, since many patients come from out of town or out of state for treatment. It is essential to convey to the floor nurses any problems encountered during the procedure that are likely to affect the patient's recovery, for example, any difficulty with the anesthetic, blood pressure stabilization, unusual bleeding, or packing of the vagina, which must remain in place to assure correct application of the radiation dose. When the patient is brought down to the clinic for removal of the radiation sources, the applicator, and the catheter, the nurse reiterates the care the patient must take to prevent postradiation bladder, vaginal, and bowel side effects, and the nurse arranges the patient's follow-up clinic visit.

CARING FOR PATIENTS TREATED BY IMMUNOTHERAPY

The body's normal surveillance system, comprised of lymphocytes and humoral factors, has in the past been able to recognize tumor cells as foreign and to keep those cells under control. When a tumor develops, this immunologic control system has been overwhelmed in some way, allowing cancer cells to multiply unchecked.[20] Patients with certain types of tumors are treated by immunotherapeutic methods in an attempt to stimulate a weakened immune system to once again regain control over tumor cells. It is postulated that tumor antigen on the tumor cell membrane elicits the production of antibodies, called blocking antibodies, which combine with receptor sites of lymphocytes, previously sensitized by tumor contact, in such a way as to inactivate or block lymphocyte-mediated interaction and destruction of tumor cells. In our clinic the nurse is responsible for carrying out several immune system survey techniques to aid in assessing the patient's immune status, and for administering the materials currently used to stimulate the host immune mechanism.

There are three immunologic survey techniques frequently used with those clinic patients treated by immunotherapy. First, the measurement of serum blocking antibody titer is done by a technician in the tumor immunology laboratory in the adjacent research center. An elevation of blocking antibody titer is indicative of tumor presence, sometimes long before tumor is clinically evident.[8] The nurse usually draws 10 ml of blood for the evaluation (a 19-gauge needle is used to prevent the fracture of blood cells and subsequent hemolysis of the sample) and injects the blood into a sterile, silicone-coated clot tube. The tube is labeled with the patient's name and is placed in the refrigerator for the technician.

Second, delayed hypersensitivity skin testing[1,19] is done to assess the patient's capacity to respond to treatment by non-specific immunotherapeutic stimulants. Using three antigens to which most people have been exposed in childhood, and purified protein derivative (PPD) of the tubercle bacillus, to which each person may or may not have been sensitized, the nurse injects these recall antigens intradermally to assess the patient's previous immune system reactivity (previous ability to be sensitized by antigens). The patient is instructed to measure the hardened (indurated) areas, where the four antigens were injected, in 48 hours. A sheet of printed instructions accompanies the verbal instructions given in the clinic; it includes a schematic diagram of the volar surfaces of each arm, with numbers 1 to 4, corresponding to the antigens administered, printed on the diagrams of the arms. In one corner of the sheet is a millimeter ruler to be used by the patient to measure the indurations, each one in perpendicular diameters. Recall antigens are injected periodically to assess whether the patient's ability to "remember" previous sensitization to antigens stays the same or diminishes, indicating indirectly whether there has been an overwhelming influence on the host immune mechanism.

Finally, to assess a patient's present ability to be sensitized to an antigen, a chemical, dinitrochlorobenzene (DNCB),[3,4] to which most people have not been sensitized, is applied to the volar surface of each forearm, a 2000 mcg. dose to the left, and a 50 mcg. dose to the right. The chemical is allowed to dry and is covered with a Telfa pad and occlusive tape. The patient is instructed to keep the forearms dry and the dressings on for 24 hours. When he removes the dressings, he begins to keep his 14-day record of the appearance of the right and left forearms, noting any redness, itching, or blistering. Again, as with the recall antigens, the nurse instructs the patient verbally, reinforcing the instructions with a printed set of the same instructions (with the patient record on the back of the sheet) regarding what to expect, what to note, and when to return the record to the clinic. From the standpoint of an immunologic survey, it is of import if the high dose site becomes red or blistered within 24 to 48 hours, begins to fade, and then flares in 10 to 14 days. This indicates to the physician that the patient is currently capable of being sensitized to a new antigen.

DNCB is also used to stimulate the production of lymphocytes. These circulating white blood cells are immunologically active against tumor cells, initiating the destruction of the tumor cells. DNCB, usually in a dose of 100 mcg./0.1 ml., is dropped directly onto superficial tumor nodules or is placed adjacent to tumor infiltrates. Systemic side effects of this treatment are infrequent but can occur because DNCB sensitization takes place in the regional lymph nodes and can cause enlargement and tenderness of the nodes.

In conjunction with the Hellström laboratory at the University of Washington, an immunotherapeutic protocol for the treatment of malignant melanoma, using plasma and Bacillus Calmette-Guérin (BCG) vaccine, has been developed.[7] For those patients selected to participate in the protocol, plasma is given every other week to provide unblocking antibodies to assist the host immune mechanism in regaining the ability to recognize and destroy tumor cells. BCG vaccine is applied on alternate weeks by scarification as a nonspecific lymphocyte stimulant.[2,6]

Each time, before plasma is administered, blood for blocking antibody titer is drawn, and then the nurse begins the plasma infusion. In patients who have known hypersensitivity with past plasma administration, diphenhydramine (Benadryl), 25 to 50 mg., is taken by the patient 30 minutes before arriving in the clinic. The hypersensitivity reaction, which is an allergic reaction, is usually manifested by the development of urticaria and sometimes facial edema. One patient progressed to a more severe anaphylactic reaction, with hypotension and respiratory distress. The reactions seem better controlled, or prevented altogether, by slow administration of the plasma (about 45 to 60 minutes) and by premedication with oral Benadryl. The patient is placed in a room close to the nursing station, is checked frequently by the nurse, and is given a bell with which to call the nurse; instructions are given to call if there is any concern, and the patient soon learns to observe the rate of flow (too fast, too slow, or plasma finished) and to observe his own reaction (development of itching or difficulty in breathing). An emergency box containing injectable Benadryl, epinephrine, aminophylline, and cortisone (as well as other emergency drugs) is kept in the workroom.

The BCG vaccine is administered to melanoma protocol patients and to other selected patients in order to stimulate, by scarification, lymphyocyte production in the region of administration.[2a] It can also be administered, in a dilute solution, intralesionally or intravenously. Scarification is accomplished in our clinic by using freshly prepared BCG in a syringe with a 21-gauge needle. The area to be scarified is cleansed with acetone to remove any oils; the needle point is then lightly and quickly drawn over the skin as the skin is held taut, breaking the skin but not deeply lacerating it. Five scratches, 5 cm. in length and 1 cm. apart, are made in one direction, and then five more scratches are made perpendicular to the first set, forming a grid pattern. The BCG vaccine is dropped onto and spread over the broken skin and then dried with the use of a hair dryer. The area is covered with plastic film and waterproof tape, and the patient is instructed to keep the area dry and the dressing on for 24 hours, at which time the dressing is to be removed and the skin washed gently. The patient is told to expect, at the most, symptoms of the flu—aching, fever, swollen regional lymph nodes, and malaise for the first 24 to 48 hours; previous BCG scars may also flare up with each new scarification.

Intralesional BCG vaccine is administered only by a physician, attendant side effects and risks being greater with intralesional injection than with superficial scarification.[18] The patient is usually hospitalized; however, the clinic nurse's responsibility to the patient lies in informing the floor nurses, by telephone or by a prominent note on the chart, that the patient has received intralesional BCG vaccine and that any one of the following may be experienced: an elevation of temperature as high as 105° F., hypotension, a dusky skin color, or convulsions. Intralesional BCG has infrequently resulted in death. The floor nurses need to be advised to monitor blood pressure, temperature, color, and state of consciousness of a patient who has received intralesional BCG vaccine that day; they need to be informed that the appearance of any of the above reactions will necessitate notification of the clinic physician on an emergency basis.

GENERAL NURSING CARE ADAPTED TO CANCER PATIENTS IN A CLINIC SETTING

Pain is more easily and efficiently controlled when at first a slightly greater than adequate amount of medication is given.[5] Then the amount is carefully adjusted, based on nursing evaluation including patient input, in doses to be given before pain again becomes aggravating enough to necessitate the patient's telling the nurse (or acknowledging to himself) that pain is present. This means that a type of schedule is maintained to make it possible for the nurse and patient to evaluate the time interval in which the patient is comfortable between analgesic doses. It should be stressed to the patient that the longer he waits between doses, to the point of becoming increasingly uncomfortable, the greater the amount of analgesic necessary to bring his pain under control again.

Saunders[15] writes, "The art of giving analgesics for continuous pain in terminal illness is to administer such drugs continually at the optimum dose level for each individual." Waiting until pain overcomes the patient, and then giving enough analgesic to relieve the pain, produce what hospital nurses frequently observe—the very uncomfortable patient who, when he receives his 15 mg. of morphine, drops off to sleep, exhausted from his struggle with pain. It is my belief that the discomfort-analgesic-sleep pattern reinforces the nurses's already cautious reticence to give adequate and more frequent small doses of analgesics. In London, at St. Joseph's Hospice, I observed that when patients were given analgesics in individualized doses once every 4 hours, no one was uncomfortable, and no one was asleep, or "knocked out" by medication. The St. Joseph's mixture is composed of drugs not available for medical use in the United States, but the principle, that of individualized doses given at regular intervals, can eliminate the discomfort-analgesic-sleep pattern, in which the quality of life is at a minimum, and thus allow patients to be free of pain and awake to carry on their daily living and planning.

With the chronic pain that some cancer patients experience, the clinic nurse needs to ask at each visit whether the patient has enough pain medication to last easily until the next visit; this inquiry at each visit not only assures the patient of an adequate supply of medication but also reduces the number of telephone calls and written prescriptions to be telephoned and then mailed, in accordance with present narcotic regulations. In addition, at each visit, the nurse evaluates, by verbal and nonverbal information, the efficacy of the patient's present analgesic; for this evaluation, the nurse needs to develop the sensitivity and skills necessary to detect pain in the person who verbalizes well-being but who has in fact a furrowed brow, a clenched fist, a fidgety bearing, or an irritated or vague affect. Of course, these signs can mean other things—for example, a delayed appointment or a dislike of the impending treatment—but detecting these nonverbal clues helps the nurse to direct questions toward the status of the patient's pain.

With narcotic analgesia comes chronic constipation. Again, by obtaining a prescription for appropriate medication, recommending bulk in the diet, and encouraging an increased fluid intake, the nurse anticipates the problem before the patient has developed it.

Some patients receiving chemotherapy or radiation therapy experience nausea and periodically take antiemetic medication. In addition, some patients take tranquilizers or muscle relaxants. Patients should be cautioned about the potentiation of their narcotic analgesics by phenothiazines and by other related compounds; on the other hand, patients can be helped to extend the effect of analgesics by the concomitant use of phenothiazines. Regardless, they need to know what to expect when combining their medications.

Although we have no nurse in the radiation area, it is appropriate whenever possible to check on those hospital patients brought down for treatment or for minor surgical procedures, to see that they are comfortable and have had adequate pain medication if needed before having left the hospital floor. If they have not, the nurse must bring to the clinic physician's attention the discomfort and obtain an order for appropriate medication.

As with pain control, assessment of present or anticipated problems with nausea, sleep, or depression is brought to the physician's attention, and appropriate intervention or medication is obtained. The patient is instructed about possible side effects and about the proper way to obtain the most benefit from the drugs.

COORDINATION AND CONTINUITY OF CARE

As mentioned earlier in the section on chemotherapy, as the nurse must develop excellent intravenous skills before administering chemotherapy, so should any laboratory technician who draws blood from cancer patients, for cancer patients' veins, particularly those of chemotherapy patients, are precious. They are *not* to be the objects of practice! The nurse lets the laboratory know that experienced persons are to do the blood drawing and also makes a note on the laboratory requisition if the patient has difficult veins. A missed venipuncture means not only a shaken patient and a possible infection or hematoma due to the patient's leukopenia or thrombocytopenia but also a lost vein for chemotherapy until the vein heals.

It is of help in the overall assessment of the patient's condition if his general appearance, personality, strength, color, and mobility are observed by the nurse on each visit. It is of little value for the nurse to assume that any change she notes in the patient is due to medication, for example, or to the progression of the tumor if that change is not brought to the physician's attention for his comparison and evaluation. A normally alert patient may come for an appointment, and the nurse may notice that he is "vague"; if this unusual vagueness is not mentioned to the physician, overmedication, an impending cerebral hemorrhage in the presence of thrombocytopenia, or developing brain metastasis might otherwise go unnoticed and unevaluated until the symptoms become more pronounced.

To personalize care, to include the patient in decisions that he *can* make about his care, as well as to promote safe nursing, the nurse should inquire about patient preference whenever possible. For example, the arm on the side of a woman's mastectomy remains sensitive to compression by a blood pressure cuff or a tourniquet; whenever possible, the other arm should be used for intravenous therapy or blood pressure monitoring. Or a person may always sleep on one side and may prefer to have an intramuscular injection known to cause local pain administered in one particular hip.

Patients are frequently admitted to the hospital from the clinic. Before telephoning the admitting office to reserve a bed, the nurse provides more complete care by obtaining specific information from the patient. Does the patient smoke? Prefer a nonsmoking roommate? Prefer (or need) a private room? Need a room with a bath for colostomy care or urinary frequency? Use oxygen? Have a low white blood cell count, necessitating absolutely that the patient not be placed with a roommate who has an infection or a cold? Some of the preference information the nurse obtains is impossible to implement, but certainly the patient who does not smoke, who will be on oxygen, or who has a low white blood cell count must be given optimum consideration for the appropriate room, and it is the nurse's responsibility to make it clear in an admitting situation when an appropriate room or roommate is mandatory for the patient's welfare.

Several clinic patients a day are admitted to the hospital for care. After having worked for several years on the medical floor that receives the majority of our clinic's patients, I have a great appreciation for the information and support the clinic nurse can give to the floor nurse. It is important to maintain communication with the hospital nurses and to bring to the physician's attention any problems the floor nurses note with each hospitalized clinic patient. It is helpful when time permits to visit the patients admitted from the clinic to the hospital to coordinate their care with the floor nurses, imparting the special knowledge of the patient and perhaps of the family. This creates in the patient a feeling of continuity about the care received.

The floor staff appreciates any teaching the clinic nurse can do in an informal way or a short interval. For example, a demonstration of BCG vaccine may be given by scarification; conduct a visual inspection of the intracavitary radiation applicators; or review what the floor nurses can expect when a patient has just received intralesional BCG vaccine, chemotherapy, plasma, or whole brain irradiation.

Patient assessment is aided when the clinic nurse relays observations about the hospitalized clinic patient to the clinic physician, who, after all, sees the patient for perhaps only 5 to 10 minutes a day. If rapport is established between the floor nurses and the clinic nurses, telephone messages about problems and needed orders can be given between physician visits to the floor, accelerating and improving patient care for the clinic patient in the hospital.

REFERENCES

1. Al-Sarrof, M., and others: Clinical immunologic responsiveness in malignant disease. 1. Delayed hypersensitivity reaction and the effect of cytotoxic drugs, Cancer 26:262-268, Aug., 1970.
2. Bast, R. C., Jr., and others: BCG and cancer (part 1), New England Journal of Medicine 290:1413-1420, June 20, 1974.
2a. Cancer immunotherapy starts from scratch, Medical World News 14:39-53, Feb. 23, 1973.
3. Catolona, W. J., and others: A method for dinitrochlorobenzene contact sensitization, New England Journal of Medicine 286:399-402, Feb. 24, 1972.
4. Chakravorty, R. C., and others: The delayed hypersensitivity reaction in the cancer patient: observations on sensitization by DNCB, Surgery 73:730-735, May 19, 1973.
5. "Getting to Know St. Joseph's Hospice" (pamphlet). Obtained from the Irish Sisters of Charity at St. Joseph's Hospice, 8 Mare Street, London, E2, England, 1972.
6. Gutterman, J. U., and others: Active immunotherapy with B.C.G. for recurrent malignant melanoma, Lancet 1: 1208-1212, June 2, 1973.
7. Hellstrom, I., and others: Destruction of cultivated melanoma cells by lymphocytes from healthy black (North American Negro) donors, International Journal of Cancer 11:116-122, 1973.
8. Hellstrom, I., and others: Sequential studies on cell-mediated tumor immunity and blocking serum activity in ten patients with malignant melanoma, International Journal of Cancer 11:280-292, 1973.
9. Hendrickson, F. R., and Browning, D.: Radiotherapy treatment for cancer: guidelines for nursing care, Journal of practical Nursing 22:18-20 passim, Feb., 1972.
10. Lowenbraun, S.: Chemotherapy of malignant disease. In Rosenfeld, M. G., editor: Manual of medical therapeutics, ed. 20, Boston, 1971, Little, Brown & Co.
11. McCorkle, M. R.: Coping with physical symptoms in metastatic breast cancer,

American Journal of Nursing **73:**1034-1038, June, 1973.

12. Rodman, M. J.: Anticancer chemotherapy. Part 1. The kinds of drugs and what they do, RN **35:**45-56, Feb., 1972.

13. Rodman, M. J.: Anticancer chemotherapy. Part 2. Against solid malignant tumors, RN **35:**61-78, March 19, 1972.

14. Rodman, M. J.: Anticancer chemotherapy. Part 3. Against leukemias and lymphomas, RN **35:**49-64, April, 1972.

15. Saunders, C.: The last stages of life, American Journal of Nursing **65:**70-75, March, 1965.

16. Shafer, K. N., and others: Medical-surgical nursing, ed. 6, St. Louis, 1975, The C. V. Mosby Co.

17. Snider, M. A.: Helpful hints on I.V.'s, American Journal of Nursing **74:**1978-1981, Nov., 1974.

18. Sparks, F. C., and others: Complications of BCG immunotherapy in patients with cancer, New England Journal of Medicine **289:**827-830, Oct. 18, 1973.

19. Sumner, D. S., and others: Depression of delayed hypersensitivity and abnormal bone scans in early cancer of the breast, British Journal of Surgery **59:**897, Nov., 1972.

20. Warner, G. A.: Immunotherapeutic approaches to cancer control, AORN **17:**71-74, May, 1973.

21. Welsh, M. S.: Comfort measures during radiation therapy, American Journal of Nursing **67:**1880, Sept., 1967.

6 Role of the nurse in antineoplastic drug research

CYNTHIA ALLISON MANTZ
GEORGE J. HILL, II

I still walk through clinics and see cancer patients with eyes full of fear. I see the cancer patient being avoided and neglected on wards. In my mind I have always questioned the "traditional" way of treating these patients. It seemed so easy for residents and staff doctors to say, "We can offer nothing except morphine." I knew there just *had* to be something else to offer, and more that could be done. That is where my commitment to become an oncology nurse began. Within the oncologic service, I work as a chemoimmunotherapy nurse.

I have found my new role to be exciting and demanding. Oncologic nursing draws from all one's resources in the areas of pharmacology, psychology, physiology, and sociology. In this chapter I will discuss the role of an oncology nurse, specifically in an institution offering solid tumor treatment and engaging in research. However, the role of the individual nurse depends on her independence and initiative, as well as her colleagues. In my position I have the opportunity to institute or change treatment in some cases.

Cancer chemotherapy is defined as the treatment of cancer with drugs, including antimetabolites, alkylating agents, antibiotics, hormones, and a broad spectrum of miscellaneous compounds. The goal of all therapy is complete control ("cure"), or palliation, which is defined as relief of pain and extension of a useful life. No longer is chemotherapy instituted only in "terminal" patients. Cancer is not, and should not be considered, a hopeless disease. Advances in the field now have given us *complete* control of tumor growth in many instances. Chemotherapy has become an acceptable method of treating cancer, thus making pretreatment evaluation necessary. Pretreatment evaluation by all oncology specialists is now considered worthwhile. Patients may now undergo surgery, radiation therapy, and/or chemotherapy at the same time; the drugs are no longer used only as a last resort.

Let us begin with a step-by-step approach to a patient who is being evaluated for chemotherapy. Referrals may be made by physicians, patients, or other nurses. Every referral is followed up by our team or by those we recommend. We begin assessment by seeing the patient. At that time a physical examination, history, blood tests, and x-ray examination are done. They are obtained for a baseline, which is important because disease processes can be evaluated through many of

68

these parameters. All information, past and present, must be obtained. After organizing all the available information, a decision is made as to what type of treatment is going to be initiated. Primarily we are involved in clinical trials of which protocols (outlines of experiments) are the guidelines. Our clinical trials evaluate methods of treatment, particularly with experimental drugs. If a patient meets the criteria for acceptance into a clinical trial, our statistics office is called and the patient is randomly assigned to a treatment group.

If the patient does not meet the requirements of the protocol, a standard recommendation is made and implemented. In many instances the nurse takes the history, recommends what can be done, asks that certain tests be obtained, and keeps records for the statistics office to analyze responses to treatment if a protocol is instituted. She not only assists in follow-up treatment but often initiates treatment. This demonstrates one of many ways in which the nurse provides a liaison between physician and patient.

At this time, side effects and prognosis are fully explained. This conference is invaluable in allaying anxiety, establishing rapport, and relaying and obtaining information. Every member of the conference has a chance to voice an opinion. We work with both the patient and the family. Our belief is that patients should be made fully aware of their diagnosis, prognosis, and treatment, and the indications for that treatment. Informed consent is obtained before therapy begins. Working with instead of working on the patient is one of our major goals. Because patients know the normal blood counts, and see their chest x-ray films, they can work actively with us in treating their disease.

Communication is essential, and here again the nurse forms the foundation by reviewing the entire treatment. Patients often say, "I did not want to bother the doctor because he's so busy, but can you explain what he meant by some of his medical talk?" Families will often come to me with financial or emotional problems that they "didn't think the doctor wanted to hear." By maintaining a concerned attitude, good rapport is established. The patient's questions are innumerable, but of greatest concern is the question, "Is the drug going to cure my cancer?" Our reply is an honest no. However, digitalis does not cure heart disease either. The next question usually is: "How will the drug affect me?" Full explanations regarding all side effects are given, and the patient knows whether he is receiving standard therapy or investigational therapy. Because questions are constantly being asked, the nurse must understand the mechanism of the action of the drugs.

CELLULAR METABOLISM

In order to understand the mechanism of action of the drugs, a background in cellular metabolism is needed (see Fig. 1).

Resting cells (not ready to divide) contain dark-staining granules called chromatin material, which is arranged in loose coils called chromosomes. Chromosomes consist of DNA (deoxyribonucleic acid), which is a double-coiled helix. The foundation, or backbone, of each DNA strand is a recurring sugar (deoxyribose)

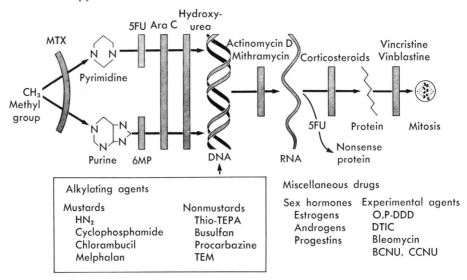

Fig. 1. Mechanism of action of commonly used chemotherapeutic agents.

and a phosphate group. The connectors of the two strands are pairs of nitrogenous bases, pyrimidines and purines. The usual purines in DNA are adenine and guanine, and the pyrimidines are thymine and cytosine. These nitrogenous bases constitute the "genetic code." DNA directs the synthesis of ribonucleic acid (RNA) on which protein is synthesized. RNA resembles DNA; however, ribose, rather than deoxyribose, is the foundation. Further, RNA contains uracil rather than thymine.

The first step in protein synthesis is the formation of messenger RNA from DNA. Enzymes are proteins, and every chemical reaction that takes place in the body is accomplished by specific enzymes. Thus DNA and RNA have the essential role in cell kinetics. Cellular organization and function are extremely complicated and incompletely understood processes. The importance of cellular growth will be stressed for the purpose of this discussion.

Groups of growing (proliferating) cells demonstrate certain phases that, taken together, constitute the cell cycle of growth and division. These phases are G_1, S, G_2, and M. Phase G_1 occurs prior to the start of DNA synthesis in which organization occurs, with the enzymes preparing for synthesis. The actual replication (synthesis) of DNA occurs in the next phase, called S, which lasts about 6 to 8 hours. After replication of DNA, further protein and RNA synthesis occurs in the G_2 phase. After this, the entire structural redesigning of the cell is accomplished in the mitotic phase.

Cell division is called mitosis, which has four parts: prophase, metaphase, anaphase, and telophase. Prophase is the stage in which two chromatids (daughter cells) form. Metaphase is the stage in which the chromatids become organized in the middle of the cell and are connected to tubules. The two chromatids separate— are pulled apart by spindle tubules—in anaphase, and are then said to be chro-

Text continued on p. 76.

Table 2. Major drugs

Drug	Usual doses	Indications	Toxicity Manifestations	Management
Antimetabolites				
5 FU (5 Fluoroura-cil; Efudex, Fluoroplex ointment)	500 to 100 mg/wk orally or IV	Gastrointestinal Breast	1. Stomatitis	1. Good oral hygiene
			2. Diarrhea	2. Do not use laxatives; determine previous bowel habits for baseline, and chart amount
			3. Nausea	3. Nausea after small frequent meals—carbonated beverage, tea, antiemetics, prochlorperazine maleate (Compazine), or chlorpromazine hydrochloride (Thorazine)
			4. Bone marrow suppression (stops when drug discontinued)	4. Check CBC
MTX (methotrexate)	2.5 mg/24 hr orally 25 mg/wk IV	Alone or in combination (MOPP) Metastatic trophoblastic disease, leukemia, lymphosarcoma, advanced unresponsive psoriasis	1. Stomatitis 2. Diarrhea 3. Dermatitis 4. Pancytopenia—resistance to infection 5. Hepatic toxicity 6. Renal failure 7. Cystitis 8. Menstrual dyfunction 9. Alopecia 10. Headache and blurred vision	Management same as 5FU NOTE: Observe for adequate renal function. Drug must be stopped immediately or if renal function deteriorates. Obtain SMA-12s, and check creatinine. Drug accumulates in tissues, especially liver, leading to higher serum levels in higher doses. Drug interacts with sulfonomides, diphenylhydantoin, antibacterials, folic-acid–containing vitamins.

Continued.

Table 2. Major drugs—cont'd

Drug	Usual doses	Indications	Toxicity Manifestations	Management
6MP (6-mer-captopurine; Purinethol)	50 to 150 mg/24 hr orally	Leukemia	1. Oral and gastroin-testinal tract ulcer-ation 2. Bone mar-row depres-sion 3. Leukopenia 4. Thombocy-topenia	1. Oral care and frequent antacids 2. Check CBC
Ara C (cytosine arabinoside, cytarabine, Cytosar)	1 to 3 mg/ kg/24 hr orally	Leukemia	1. Bone marrow depression 2. Nausea and vomiting 3. Megaloblas-tosis 4. Leukopenia 5. Thrombocy-topenia	1. Check CBC 2. Antiemetics
Hydroxyurea (Hydrea)	20 to 30 mg/kg/24 hr orally	Leukemia	1. Nausea 2. Bone mar-row depres-sion	1. Antiemetics 2. Check RBC
Mitotic inhibitors Vincristine (Oncovin) Vinblastine (Velban)	1 to 2 mg/ wk IV 5 to 10 mg/ wk IV	Combination therapy Combination therapy	1. Neuropa-thy 2. Paresthesia 3. Bone mar-row suppres-sion 4. Neurotox-icity	1. Watch tendon re-flexes 2. Watch for constipation
Antibiotics Adriamycin (doxorubicin)	0.4 to 0.6 mg/kg/ wk 60 mg/M² every 3 weeks	Breast cancer Combination therapy	1. Stomatitis 2. Pancyto-penia 3. Cardiac ab-normalities 4. Alopecia— 5. Urine may be red	1. As with 5FU 2. As with 5FU 3. Electrocardio-gram and CPK should be monitored 4. Advise patient that alopecia will surely occur

Table 2. Major drugs—cont'd

Drug	Usual doses	Indications	Toxicity Manifestations	Management
Dactinomycin (actinomycin D; Cosmegen)	0.5 to 1 mg/ wk IV Also given in more intensive courses	Miscellaneous cancers, and in combination with other drugs	1. Stomatitis 2. Pancyto- penia 3. Alopecia 4. Acne in males	As with adriamycin Advise patient that alopecia will probably occur
Mithramycin (Mithricin)	0.5 mg/kg IV q.o.d. and 4 doses	Cancer of testis	1. Hypocalce- mia 2. Thrombocy- topenia 3. Phlebitis 4. Epistaxis— may be first sign of toxicity	Fatal sx have oc- curred suddenly
Bleomycin (Blenoxane)	15 to 30 mg 2 or 3x/ wk IV	Cancer of testis Cancer of larynx, head, and neck Lymphomas	1. Pulmonary fibrosis 2. Fever 3. Dermatitis	1. Chest x-ray films
Streptozotocin	12.5 mg/kg/ wk	Pancreatic islet cell tumors	1. Nausea 2. Vomiting	Still under investi- gational use
Hormones Corticosteroids, Cortisone- acetate Prednisone- dexametha- sone	25 to 37.5 mg/24 hr orally 0.75 to 16 mg/24 hr orally	Cancer of prostate Brain tumors	1. Cushing's syndrome 2. Fluid reten- tion 3. Hyperten- sion 4. Osteoporosis 5. Susceptibil- ity to infection	1. Check electrolytes 2. Check BP
Estrogens— Premarin, DES, TACE	1 to 5 mg/ 24 hr (males) 5 to 15 mg/ 24 hr (elderly females)	Cancer of prostate Metastatic cancer of breast	1. Fluid reten- tion 2. Cardiac failure 3. Feminiza- tion	1. Check electrolytes 2. ECG
Androgens— fluoxy- mesterone (Halotestin), calusterone (Methosarb), testalactone Teslac	100 mg 3x/ wk 30 mg/24 hr 200 mg/24 hr	Metastatic cancer of breast	1. Mascu- liniza- tion 2. Nausea 3. Fluid reten- tion 4. Jaundice	1. Check electrolytes

Continued.

Table 2. Major drugs—cont'd

Drug	Usual doses	Indications	Toxicity	
			Manifestations	**Management**
Progestins—medroxy-progesterone acetate (Provera, Depo-Provera) hydroxy-progesterone caproate (Delalutin)	2500 to 5000 mg/wk	Cancer of endo-metrium Cancer of kidney	1. Susceptibility to infection 2. Euphoria or depression 3. Cushing's syndrome 4. Peptic ulcers 5. Osteoporosis 6. Myopathy 7. Hyperglycemia 8. Virilization 9. Thrombo-embolism	1. Avoid contact with infectious organisms 2. Assess mental and emotional status 4. Bland diet 6. Assess muscle weakness
Alkylating agents Cyclophospha-mide (Cytoxan)	50 to 150 mg/24 hr orally 500 to 1000 mg/wk IV	Lymphosarcoma Leukemia Cystadenocarci-noma of ovary Breast cancer Lung cancer	1. Hemor-rhagic cystitis 2. Nausea and vomiting 3. Alopecia	1. Encourage 2 to 3 quarts of fluid per 24 hours; early with break-fast 2. Management same as 5FU
Thio-Tepa	30 to 60 mg IV—can be given by intra-pleural or intraperi-toneal route	1. Cystadenocarci-noma of ovary 2. Lymphoma 3. Breast cancer	1. Pancyto-penia	1. Check blood counts frequently and adjust dos-age accordingly
Mechloretha-mine hydrochlo-ride (nitrogen mustard; Mustargen)	Initially 0.4 mg/kg IV or as daily doses of 0.1 mg/kg for 2 to 4 days IV, or a single intra-cavitary dose	Pleural effusions	1. Nausea and vomiting 2. Irritating to tissues 3. Permanent bone mar-row depres-sion	1. Give Thorazine or Compazine 30 to 50 minutes before adminis-tration 2. Prevent extrava-sation or drug coming into con-tact with skin 3. Watch blood counts carefully

Table 2. Major drugs—cont'd

Drug	Usual doses	Indications	Toxicity	
			Manifestations	**Management**
Melphalan(L-phenylala-nine mustard, L-PAM; Alkeran)	2 to 4 mg tablets orally per per 24 hours for 5 days repeated every 6 weeks	Breast cancer	1. Nausea after leukopenia and throm-bocytopenia	1. Check course frequently
Procarbazine (Matulane, Natulan)	50 mg/24 hr orally	Combination therapy MOPP Hodgkin's disease	1. Nausea and vomiting 2. Neurotoxic-ity	1. Antiemetics
Busulfan (Myleran)	4.8 mg/24 hr orally	Chronic leukemia	1. Bone mar-row depres-sion	1. Check RBC
Miscellaneous drugs Nitrosoureas, CCNU, BCNU	100 to 200 mg/M² every 4 to 6 weeks	Glioblastomas	1. Nausea and vomiting 2. Bone mar-row depres-sion	1. Antiemetics 2. Check RBC
Quinacrine (Atabrine) Chloquine (Aralen	500 to 1000 mg into affected pleural cavity	Pleural effusion	1. Fever 2. Malaise 3. Severe vomiting	1. Check tempera-ture 3. Antiemetics
BCG vaccine*	1 ml intra-lesionally, orally, or intrader-mally by scarifica-tion	Peripheral tumors, malignant melanoma	1. Fever 2. Nausea and vomiting	1. Check tempera-ture 2. Antiemetics
DTIC (dimeth-yltriazenomi-dazole car-boxamide dacarbazine)	IV push Alone 4.5 mg/kg over 10-day pe-riod	Combination therapy Alone for malig-nant melanoma	1. Same as for BCG with flulike syn-drome	1. Same as for BCG 2. Burns during injection. Avoid extravasation

*See pp. 62 and 63.

mosomes. Telophase is the last stage of mitosis. The cell then actually divides, forming two new cells, each with forty-six chromosomes. Some cells, such as bone marrow, skin, and gastrointestinal cells, are constantly undergoing mitosis. However, central nervous system cells never divide after the organs are completely formed. The problem of cancer begins when an abnormal, uncontrolled cellular growth occurs *without the need for function.* If unchecked, these cells have the potential to injure vital organs, spread throughout the body, and cause death.

Table 2 organizes information about the various drugs used in cancer chemotherapy. Nursing interventions have been included.

TUMORS—CHOICE OF THERAPY

In an evaluation of a patient for chemotherapy, many factors are considered. The first consideration, of course, is the source of tumor or primary lesions.

Colorectal system

Adenocarcinoma of the colorectal system is usually treated with 5FU intravenously, and 17% to 30% of patients respond; 5FU or 5FUDR can also be given arterially through the hepatic artery. If there is no response, the patient has a slight chance of responding with alkylating agents such as cyclophosphamide (Cytoxan) or Alkeran. Other tumors of the colorectal system can be cloacogenic (transitional cell) or epidermoid, and these types may respond to bleomycin and BCNU.

Gastrointestinal system

The tumors arising from the gastrointestinal system are difficult to treat due to the fact that objectively measurable disease is rarely seen. Esophageal carcinoma is a poor responder to any treatment. Squamous cell carcinoma may respond to bleomycin, methotrexate, or 5FU. Adenocarcinoma of the stomach is treated with 5FU, and again a 30% response rate is seen. Adenocarcinoma of the pancreas is treated with 5FU as first choice. However, additional agents such as BCNU, Tubercidin, and streptozotocin can be used in combination with 5FU. Small bowel, bile duct, and gallbladder with adenocarcinoma are treated with 5FU, and approximately 30% respond.

Lung

Oat cell carcinoma may respond to treatment with cyclophosphamide (Cytoxan) or with a combination of cyclophosphamide, methotrexate, and vincristine. A response rate of 20% to 50% is seen. Epidermoid carcinoma and adenocarcinoma rarely respond to any chemotherapy. However, the previously mentioned drugs, as well as nitrogen mustard, can be given for a trial.

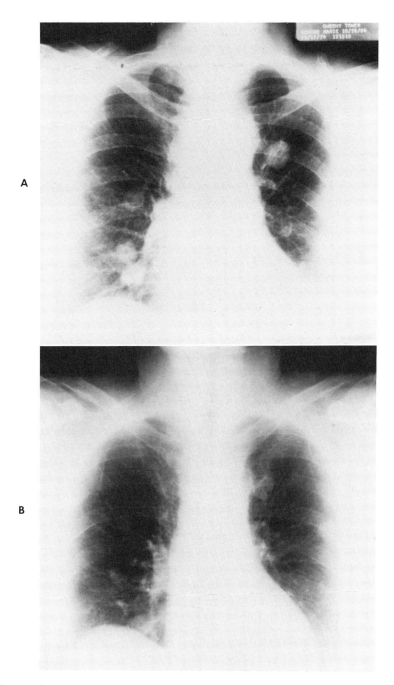

Fig. 2. A, The nurse can evaluate chest films. In this case patient has metastatic angio-sarcoma. **B,** Patient was treated with adriamycin, and response was seen 2 weeks after beginning of therapy.

Breast

All types of breast cancer are treated with one or more of five specific drugs: 5FU, methotrexate, vincristine, cyclophosphamide, and prednisone. Research has shown that when all five drugs are used, 60% to 90% of the tumors respond. However, if one of the agents is used (excluding prednisone), a 20% to 30% response rate is seen. Adriamycin also appears to be useful in the treatment of breast cancer and is the drug of choice in metastatic angiosarcoma (Fig. 2).

HOW TO ADMINISTER AND WHEN TO ADMINISTER

Although it is imperative for the nurse to know about the complexity of the drugs, she must be flexible enough to assume her role in many other aspects. It is archaic to believe that the nurse cannot accept a major responsibility for the care of the patient. I find it extremely challenging to be able to handle a patient in a diversified way. For example, Mr. H. is a 50-year-old man with carcinoma that metastasized from the colon to the lung. He was referred to us by a local physician. Initially we saw the patient and developed a treatment plan. From that point on, I became Mr. H.'s nurse, social worker, and counselor, as well as his advocate. Weekly his injections were given by his local physician, and I would see him on a monthly basis. At that time I would evaluate his chest x-ray film, measure his lesions, review his blood counts and carcinogenic embryonic antigen level, and take an interim history. After my assessment was made, I would recommend a change in his dose if necessary or another drug if the lesions were not responding. My assessments were reviewed by our staff oncologist, and the plan was then transmitted to the local physician. One month later, he presented with an acute pain in his right leg. I obtained x-ray films and saw a lytic lesion in the right femur. At that time I called a radiation oncologist and explained the patient's history and present problem. The oncologist in turn evaluated the patient and decided to irradiate the leg. In this situation, as with many others, the nurse plays a vital role in active treatment of the patient and thus must be astute enough to know when and why other therapy should be instituted.

Usually a 6-week trial will reveal how the disease is being affected by the drug. In some cases, especially in patients who have no objective parameter to evaluate, a subjective assessment must be made. Knowing each patient is imperative. For example, I can greet Mrs. S. by saying, "Good morning, how have you been?" Her facial expression tells me so much about her previous week. Since the physician is unable to see individual patients at each visit, the nurse is in an advantageous position when evaluating patient response. What one individual may think insignificant (such as weight loss) is very important with regard to the disease process. Accurate, careful patient care notes must be kept. Drugs can be changed when an adequate trial has been completed and the disease continues to progress.

If the disease appears to be under control, of course there would be no reason to interfere with the treatment. In many cases tumor cells become resistant, and the drugs are no longer effective. There is not always an easy "next step" in treatment. Each individual case takes careful planning with regard to how debilitated the patient has become due to the previous ineffective therapy or how his blood counts have tolerated treatment. At this point supportive care is essential because patients become fearful and ask: "Why is my drug going to be changed? Have you given up?" The nurse may be the determining factor in keeping the patient from having either an overly optimistic attitude or a fatalistic outlook.

In summary, the role of the nurse in antineoplastic drug research is not limited to the functions discussed in this chapter. Because of continuing research and the development of new techniques, the role will constantly grow and change. Contrary to the constant question asked of me, "Isn't your job depressing?", I find it rewarding in many ways. A cancer patient is a special patient with many complex needs. My role is intriguing and challenging, but it becomes more than just dealing with humans—it is being human.

REFERENCES

1. Cline, M. J.: Cancer chemotherapy, vol. I, Philadelphia, 1971, W. B. Saunders Co.
2. Greenwald, E. S., editor: Cancer chemotherapy, ed. 2, Flushing, N. Y., 1973, Medical Examination Publishing Co.
3. Cole, W.: Chemotherapy of cancer, Philadelphia, 1970, Lea & Febiger.
4. Hill, G. J., editor: Outpatient surgery, Philadelphia, 1973, W. B. Saunders Co.

7 Radiation therapy

KATHLEEN M. THANEY
JOSEPHINE KELLY CRAYTOR
JANET ALMETER McNALLY

Radiation therapy is one of the three major modalities used to treat malignant diseases. Treatment is designed to cure a malignancy when this seems possible or, when cure appears impossible, to prevent or relieve distressing symptoms of the disease. Both objectives of therapy are important. Cure is, of course, highly valued, but palliation becomes very important to the individual who tries to cope with pain, threatened obstruction of a body tube, a necrotic lesion, dyspnea, or any of a number of symptoms that may be associated with malignant disease. In general, treatment for cure is more vigorous and more difficult for the individual to tolerate than is palliative therapy. Members of the patient group treated for cure tend to be at an earlier stage in the course of their disease, to have had fewer insults to their body defenses, to be somewhat younger, and to be more open to hope. Even so, dealing with intensive therapy can be enervating and discouraging, and it requires supportive help and clear, thorough instruction.

During a course of therapy every effort is made to promote comfort and peace of mind, maintain function, prevent complications, and encourage interaction among patients, family members, and the helping professional staff.

The nature of ionizing radiation, its actions, the rationale for its use, and many of the specific measures used to deal with local reactions to therapy have been discussed elsewhere. Radiation protection has also been covered. This chapter will focus on some of the concepts important to an understanding of the rationale for the use of radiation therapy, on some observations made during a recent study designed to identify patients at risk of psychosocial problems during and/or after radiation therapy, and, finally, on general aspects of nursing care during therapy, using an interpersonal model.

PRINCIPLES OF RADIATION THERAPY

In a discussion of the use of ionizing radiation as a major modality of cancer treatment, the question often arises as to how radiation actually works to eradicate tumor cells but spares normal tissue. Much of this information comes to us from the radiobiologic laboratory and has had a significant effect on new treatment policies.

The curative effect of radiation therapy depends on the ability of cells to repair sublethal damage. The term *mean lethal dose* denotes the amount of radiation that delivers an average of one lethal injury per cell in an irradiated volume. Since mean lethal dose refers to the average, this means that some cells receive more than one lethal injury, whereas others receive less, and some receive none. The mean lethal dose for both tumor and normal cells is estimated to be equal.

Despite the fact that the mean lethal dose for normal and tumor cells is the same, the difference lies in the ability of normal cells to repair sublethal injury more quickly and efficiently than malignant cells. The fractionation of the radiation dose allows time for the repair of normal tissue. For example, a patient undergoing mantle radiation for Hodgkin's disease receives 1000 rads in five fractions (200 rads/24 hr) a week. Since fractionation or sublethal damage favors normal cells as opposed to tumor cells, the number of tumor cells surviving at the end of the week is progressively smaller than the number of normal cells. Finally, at the end of therapy, if a sufficient number of mean lethal doses can be applied, less than one tumor cell is left, and the patient is cured. Although the normal cells have been damaged, there are a sufficient number of normal cells left to completely reconstitute the tissues functionally. These damaged cells may cause the patient some discomfort, depending on the anatomic site being treated, but the major side effects will disappear as the tissues regain normal functioning.[1]

Another important concept of radiation is that well-oxygenated tumors are more radiosensitive than hypoxic tumors. Again fractionation becomes important, since, as it destroys tumor cells that are closer to capillary systems, hypoxic cells become exposed to a supply of oxygen and become more radiosensitive.

A third important concept involves the cellular kinetics of tumor systems. Tumor systems involve differentiated fractions and clonogenic fractions. The latter fraction is the only part that undergoes mitosis and produces new cells. A tumor system with mainly differentiated cells grow slowly, and although mean lethal doses of irradiation may be given, it may be some time before a change in the tumor size is seen, since these cells die by aging. On the contrary, in a tumor system consisting of mainly clonogenic cells there may be a rapid reduction of tumor size in response to a few fractions of radiation. A clonogenic cell that has received a dose of lethal radiation does not die until it goes through the mitotic cycle, and time of death depends on the mitotic rate of the cell system. As a result, one may see a dramatic response and reduction in size of a rapidly growing lymphoma in 3 or 4 days, whereas there may be no detectable size difference in a well-differentiated adenocarcinoma of the lung until a month after the completion of radiation therapy.

A final principle and limiting factor based on sublethal repair is the concept of normal tissue tolerance. No doubt all tumor cells could be eradicated with ionizing radiation. However, the dose of radiation required to do so is often far above tolerance of the normal surrounding tissues, and death will result from complications of treatment. The radiotherapist must be careful not to exceed these limits.

The nurse working in a radiation therapy unit can utilize these principles in caring for patients in a variety of ways. The mere understanding of the fractionation schedule allows the nurse to anticipate that 6 weeks of treatment may present problems to the patient in regard to transporation, babysitters, and lost time from work or school. Thoughtful preliminary interviewing and scheduling can often allow for such problems. The social worker often helps with financial assistance. The nurse who understands the physiologic effect of radiation can anticipate predictable side effects and play a large role in educating the patient on how to care for them. Since side effects rarely occur in the first 2 weeks of treatment, the nurse should closely monitor the patient. Side effects vary according to the anatomic site, and the nurse should be alerted to which ones the patient should expect and should help work through appropriate health care measures when they occur.

Problems concerning adequate hydration and nutrition are a continual challenge for the nurse in the radiotherapy department, since many patients experience anorexia in addition to specific side effects of therapy.

Currently there is more of a trend toward the use of combined modalities—specifically, the use of chemotherapy with radiation therapy in diseases such as oat cell carcinoma. The nurse must also be aware of the side effects of the drug and support the patient during periods of intensive combined therapy.

Fortunately with the advent of supervoltage therapy, skin reactions are nearly nonexistent except when they are purposely intended, as in the treatment of breast carcinoma. However, care should be given to properly instruct patients in good skin care.

OBSERVATIONS OF PSYCHOSOCIAL PROBLEMS

Although the data from a recent study by the Psychosocial Group at the University of Rochester Cancer Center are not yet available, many observations were made that seem useful in understanding the individual's experience during radiation therapy. There is no doubt that this experience can be very stressful for patients. Our work with patients seems to suggest that there are certain periods during the treatment process that are particularly difficult. Foremost among them is the first, or consultation, visit, during which the patient is introduced to a wide variety of experiences, explanations, and expectations, most of which may be totally unknown. Added to this is the course of events that led to referral to the radiation oncology department. What has happened to the patient prior to arrival, what information has been given about the disease, and what meaning this information has for the patient personally profoundly affect the response to this initial visit.

It is frequently difficult to obtain an objective report of exactly what patients have been told about their condition. However, even more significant in terms of intervention is the patients' understanding of the information given and their interpretation of its implications. A few simple questions such as, "How did you learn that you would be receiving radiation therapy?" can often open discussion of these issues. Being attuned to the manner in which patients recount their history, the terminology they use, and the circumstances surrounding the diagnosis can provide added information on how they are dealing with their disease. At times a question such as, "What thoughts went through your mind when you found the lump?" can be especially valuable in learning more about the fears, fantasies, or stereotyped images that patients may have. Of course, many patients may not reveal their thoughts and feelings with any depth at this point, but observing what they say and sometimes what they do not say, as well as their general manner with staff and family, can be valuable indicators of the level of stress they are experiencing and the amount of immediate and ongoing individual support they may need.

Many patients ask numerous questions during their first visit, not only about their treatment, but also about their condition. These questions should be carefully answered, but care should be given not to give more information than the patient is ready to handle. Often emotional acceptance does not keep pace with intellectual understanding, and the patient's quest for information may be a way of dealing with anxiety. In this case, overly detailed explanations may raise more anxiety than they alleviate. It is often best to give a general explanation in response to each question and then provide the opportunity to pursue the issue or drop it as the patient wishes.

Other patients indicate in various ways that they know nothing about what is wrong with them, even when objectively this information has been given to them. Although somewhat frustrating to deal with, this type of response is understandable in terms of the patient's initial sense of shock and disbelief at what is happening, and the need to handle anxiety by minimizing or even temporarily denying the diagnosis. When a patient's defenses are this high, merely repeating information is not only ineffective but may further increase anxiety. Rather, efforts to establish a relationship of trust while gradually exploring and helping the patient to verbalize fears and to deal with one issue at a time, can do much to aid the patient in keeping anxiety within manageable limits until an ability to relate more directly to the realities of the situation is acquired.

There are also other points during the treatment process at which the patient may be particularly anxious or uncomfortable. Even with adequate preparation, most patients report being "nervous" on the day they are to be treated for the first time, and describe a sense of uncertainty as to what they will experience. Many have said they had been told that there would be no pain or sensation involved, but that they needed to experience the treatment themselves before they could be sure about it.

Another source of potential stress for the patient occurs if the treatment plan must be modified or the period of therapy extended for any reason. Often the patient interprets this as a negative sign or becomes discouraged at the prospect of coming for a longer period. Much of this response can be avoided by a general explanation at the beginning of treatment. The patient should have some idea of how many treatments to expect but should also be aware that the actual number may be adjusted somewhat as the physician assesses the response to therapy.

The end of the treatment period may also be difficult for some patients, not only because side reactions and symptoms may be more troublesome at this time, but also because it represents a loss of daily contact with the staff, which may be very important in maintaining a sense of security. Reassuring the patient that the department can be called if any question arises can be very helpful.

Many patients report feeling uneasy at the time of each follow-up visit to the department, wondering if the physician might "find something else." Others have said that they relive their treatment experience in thought and memory before each follow-up visit and find it difficult to be reminded of things they would rather avoid.

Throughout the treatment course patients are very much affected by the attitudes and reactions of their families and friends. When a supportive relationship exists, the patient's capacity for tolerating therapy is often strengthened. On the other hand, many families, themselves subject to personal fears and cultural attitudes about cancer, find it difficult to deal with the situation or to know how to help. Often they, too, need an opportunity to vent their feelings and frustrations and to receive both information and guidance in understanding and responding to the patient's spoken and unspoken needs.

Sometimes insight into how a patient has negotiated an experience can be best gained after the experience is over, since openness about his reactions may be facilitated when the immediacy of the situation is past. When interviewed 3 to 5 months after treatment was completed, some patients indicated that they could not remember much of what had happened during treatment, which indicates that their stress level was such that forgetting was the most comfortable adaptation. Others spoke of their need for explanation of, and preparation for, what to expect at each point in treatment, and emphasized their importance in alleviating anxiety and helping to maintain a sense of control.

In identifying what was most difficult during the treatment experience, some patients focused on matters of personal inconvenience, such as waiting for treatment or arranging daily transportation. Others spoke of the resultant change in their lives, such as loss of independence or inability to work. Only a few patients identified the most difficult aspect as learning that they had cancer and realizing what their condition might mean for them. Apparently, different patients integrate and deal with the experience of diagnosis and treatment at different levels, and they may focus their concern on one or another aspect of the experience as a way of dealing with overwhelming threat. Other patients state that the treatment experience was not a difficult one for them, and they deny that it has had any lasting impact on their lives. To what extent these various reactions may be adaptive for the patient and to what extent they may facilitate or inhibit response to treatment require further research so that appropriate intervention can be initiated when necessary.

DEVELOPING A MODEL FOR NURSING CARE

In the attempt to develop a model appropriate for a clinical specialist in oncologic nursing, it is necessary to remember that the nursing care of patients during radiation therapy involves helping patients and their families deal with the problems caused by malignant disease—those caused by intensive therapy used to treat the disease and by the fact that the diagnosis of "cancer" is life-threatening and requires that the patient and the family go through a difficult process of adaptation. It is also helpful to remember that to be effective in this specialized care, nurses need to understand and work through their own feelings about cancer, to be comfortable in their knowledge about radiation therapy, and to be convinced of the value of the treatment to the patient, as well as the worth of the patient being treated.

Almost any individual coming to a radiation therapy department for evaluation is in a period of crisis and is faced with either the initial diagnosis of cancer or evidence of recurrent disease. Either of these situations fits the definition of crisis as an upset in the steady state in which the habitual problem-solving activities of the individual are not adequate to restore previous balance.[2] The nurse may be the person best able to help the individual clarify the situation, begin to identify resources, and try to deal with reality. Only by careful listening can the nurse evaluate the amount of anxiety the individual is experiencing, the accuracy of the patient's knowledge of the disease, the stage of adapting to all the changes that will occur, and the methods being used to cope with the stresses. Since the individual is treated daily over a period of 4 to 7 weeks, it is possible for the nurse to validate impressions, update an initial assessment of the patient periodically, and alter methods of intervening.

When the individual first comes for treatment, it is necessary to give very specific explanations of what will happen, the participation expected of a patient, and who will answer questions or talk about the situation. Although the crisis situation means that the patient is ready to learn, he may be unable to remember directions or to take responsibility for self-care until anxiety is reduced to a manageable level. Assurances and directions may have to be repeated daily until the patient finds that the treatments *are* painless, that people do care, that coping is possible, and that what the staff has said does make sense. As the individual is ready to assume more responsibility, information can be given about skin care, diet, rest, mouth care, or whatever specific measures are appropriate to prevent complications of therapy and keep side effects to a minimum. Certain general care measures will apply in most treatment settings.[3] Each center will have certain preferred procedures, and teaching should conform to them.

The teaching of self-care measures as simple, easily carried out, and logical in relation to the effects of radiation is important, not only to assure that the patient is receiving the most comfortable course of therapy possible, but also to provide clear evidence that the patient can take positive action to affect, in some small way, the course of events, emphasizing the importance of active participation in treatment.[4,5]

There is great variation in whether or not and how actively individual patients are able to become involved, and there are differences in the stage of treatment at which they are able to participate in deciding aspects of their own care. Fink's model of crisis and motivation is useful to nurses who are trying to understand patient behavior and to plan appropriate care. Fink[6] points out that the individual crisis is made up of four stages: shock, defensive retreat, acknowledgment, and adaptation. During the shock and defensive retreat phases, the patient tries to promote "safety," and any attempts to urge forward movement are frustrated. During the acknowledgment phase, growth needs emerge along with the continuing need for safety. If safety needs are met, then growth is possible. During the period of adaptation, growth needs dominate, and it is a time to help the individual accomplish things never before possible.

The idea of nursing as an interpersonal process leading to learning and growth, proposed by Peplau[7] many years ago, is still an exciting and viable one. Understanding the stages in adaptation to loss or to threatened loss makes acceptance of patient delay and vacillation easier and reinforces the confidence of the nurse in the principles of growth and learning. As patients develop confidence in their own ability to manage the course of radiation and to do things they never tried before, their confidence in themselves as a functioning, competent person and their trust in the helping people with whom they are working both increase. Even during bad days when evidence of persisting disease is found, open communication will help.[8] Assurance can be given that it is all right to be angry that eating is a chore when it should be a pleasure, or that inertia and fatigue make even small projects difficult. Expressing such problems makes them less frightening and helps the patient to realize that it is possible to deal with them.

Even if patients resist the idea of joining a therapy group or a discussion group, they may be drawn into interactions with other patients in which their recent and difficult experience can be shared in a way that gives the experience and the patient importance. Assuring a novice that one can manage therapy, can change eating habits, and can deal with a dry mouth, a sore throat, or a patch of alopecia helps to make experienced patients value their knowledge and view themselves as helping persons.

Most individuals treated by radiation are living outside the hospital, and most continue in their usual home setting. The involvement of family members in the helping process is easier when the nurse can meet with them at intervals during therapy and when the patient returns for follow-up. Just as patients may at times assume a helping role, family members can learn to be very effective helpers. A helping relationship is based on "the ability to respond accurately to another person's experience and the ability to draw effectively from one's own experience."[9] The supportive approach of the nurse as she uses the helping skills of attending, responding, initiating action, and communicating helps set the tone for patient and family. The approach applies equally well to the support of growth and recovery, and to the promotion of comfort and acceptance in a period of decline.

The nurse caring for patients during radiation therapy and in long-term follow-up has the opportunity to establish an effective helping relationship, using a model of interpersonal interaction as the basis for practice. Help and support provided during such crisis periods can result in patient and family growth and can influence how patient and family deal with the whole experience of cancer.

REFERENCES

1. Holland, J. F., and Frei, E., III, editors: Cancer medicine, Philadelphia, 1973, Lea & Febiger.
2. Rapaport, L.: The state of crisis: some theoretical considerations. In Parad, H., editor: Crisis intervention: selected readings, New York, 1955, Family Service Association of America, p. 24.
3. Craytor, J. D., and Fass, M.: The nurse and cancer patient, Philadelphia, 1970, J. B. Lippincott Co., pp. 133-166.
4. Johnson, J. E.: Approaches to the study of nursing questions and the development of nursing science: effects of structuring patients' expectation on their reactions to threatening events, Nursing Research **21:** 499-504, Nov.-Dec., 1972.
5. Tryon, P. A., and Leonard, R. F.: Giving the patient an active role. In Skipper, J. K., and Leonard, R. C., editors: Social interaction and patient care, Philadelphia, 1965, J. B. Lippincott Co., pp. 120-127.
6. Fink, St. L.: Crisis and motivation: a theoretical model, Archives of Physical Medicine and Rehabilitation **48:**592-597, Nov., 1967.
7. Peplau, H.: Interpersonal relations in nursing, New York, 1952, G. P. Putnam's Sons, p. 16.
8. Craytor, J. K.: Talking with Persons who have cancer, American Journal of Nursing **69:**744-748, April, 1969.
9. Carkhuff, R. R.: The art of helping, Amherst, Mass., 1972, Human Resources Development Press, Introduction.

ADDITIONAL READINGS

Ackerman, L.: The pathology of radiation effect of normal and neoplastic tissue, The American Journal of Roentgenology **114:** 447-459, March, 1972.
Fletcher, G.: Textbook of radiotherapy, Philadelphia, 1974, Lea & Febiger.
Tubiana, M.: The kinetics of tumor cell proliferation and radiotherapy, The British Journal of Radiology **44:**325-347, May, 1971.

ASSESSMENT FORM: RADIOTHERAPY AND HODGKIN'S DISEASE

Name
Age
Diagnosis   **Sex**   **Marital status**
Onset

Laparotomy or surgery performed
Previous laboratory tests and blood work

Present status of Hodgkin's disease

Lymph nodes should be palpated
Lumps present: location, size, mobility and adherence, shape, consistency
General strength
Appetite
Psychologic independence or dependence

Status during radiation therapy

CBC, bone marrow, electrolytes, body temperature
Skin reaction: red pigmentation, clothing, flaking and itching, wound healing, tenderness, edema, loss of hair
Gastrointestinal changes: cramping, tenderness, diarrhea, changes in electrolytes, nausea and vomiting

Status postradiation therapy

Respiratory changes: sputum production, rate & depth, cough
Circulatory changes: ↑heart rate, ↑fatigue, malaise, chest pain, SGOT, SGPT, CPK, LDH
Muscle changes: joint pain, fatigue, weakness, LDH, CPK
Psychologic effects: depression and dependence
Artificial menopause
Impotence
Gastrointestinal changes: loss of taste, salivation, dysphagia, ↑or↓ in motility, changes in electrolytes, K+ or Na+, anorexia

8 Radiotherapy and Hodgkin's disease

ANNETTE R. TEALEY

The nurse who has perused the literature on Hodgkin's disease is aware of the broad attention and study this disease has gained since it was first described by Thomas Hodgkin in 1832. Fortunately the disease is yielding its hold to the efforts of intensive study of therapy approaches to the point where the 5-year survival figure, when all stages and all cases are combined, is approximately 80%. The progress is related to increased knowledge of the spread of the disease; better histologic classification; the use of lymphangiography and laparotomy to more specifically define the parameters of disease involvement (staging); the development of effective chemotherapy; and large-scale studies that help to establish guidelines for the use of radiation, chemotherapy, or their combination in large medical centers with the necessary sophisticated equipment and personnel skill.

One major aspect of advances in control of this disease has been the development of improved radiotherapy equipment, techniques, and treatment plans. Radiotherapy is given in daily, fractionated doses over a period of weeks. During these weeks of treatment the patients have varying but rather predictable needs. To be of value to the patient, the nurse must understand the basics of radiotherapy and the expected reactions. This chapter is not intended to supplant the very necessary reading of the medical literature on the clinical and pathologic evaluation, staging, and treatment modalities for Hodgkin's disease.

The purpose is, however, to give some background information about radiotherapy treatment for this disease and to focus primarily on the patient's reactions to such treatment. The term "patient reactions" as used in this chapter will encompass the broad range of physical symptoms and effects of the radiation, as well as the response the individual makes behaviorally to these symptoms. Nursing input can be made at both points and can significantly affect patient comfort, both physiologic and psychologic. Unfortunately, the establishment of clear-cut relationships between nursing intervention and patient reactions remains in the future. I am therefore speaking from a practice base, not from an experimentally documented foundation. The new nursing role that is described is one that has far-reaching potential for care if it is refined and utilized.

In summary, this chapter will include a description of the population, an explanation of the radiotherapy treatment situation, and a review of patient reactions, as well as a discussion of the nurse's role in the care of the patient with Hodgkin's disease who is receiving radiotherapy.

Hodgkin's disease affects the young adult, with a peak in incidence occurring between the ages of 15 and 40 years. In addition, there is the characteristic rise in incidence as age rises to another peak in the seventies.[7] The disease is more prevalent among males. The American Cancer Society statistics point out that in 1974, of the 6900 estimated new cases, 4100 will be males and 2800 will be females. This is a male-female ratio of approximately 1.5:1.[1]

Hodgkin's disease was estimated to account for only 1% of all cancer deaths and only 1% of all new cancer cases in 1974. Yet because of its high incidence during the early decades of life, much attention has been focused on it. Fortunately, also, the character of the disease and concentrated efforts at improving treatment have spurred interest and hope for even better control.

The diagnosis of Hodgkin's disease during the most productive years of a person's life has far-reaching social and psychologic implications. To most people, adulthood entails work, marriage, parenthood, and establishing oneself in the life of a community. Perlman, in a book entitled *Persona: Social Role and Personality,*[9] addresses these social roles and the dynamics of change in adulthood. She states that work, at its least, can be rewarding because it links one to others with the common characteristics of age, sex, and status, and because it provides a social identity—a function recognized in society. She also speaks of its value in stabilizing and ordering habits of daily living. At its best, work is the means by which a person comes to know and find pleasure in his own effectiveness, competence, and worth. Being unable to work or limited in capacity has varying implications. To one young person it may mean a welcome escape from a boring, meaningless job. As time goes on, the inactivity can lead to boredom and feelings of being cut off from others who still are busy with the daily routine of work. To another, the illness and time involved in receiving appropriate treatment seriously interferes with daily life and work. Expectations for completing educational preparation in order to enter the job market are frequently disrupted in this young age group. Finding out one month before the end of the semester that one has Hodgkin's disease can mean a total negation of the preceding months of effort and study.

Marriage or a close personal relationship, another hallmark of young adulthood, is infinitely complex, and in every couple one will find variations of relationship, duties, and satisfactions. Though marriage in the United States is purported to be made and maintained for love, there are many other forces and considerations. Perlman includes the following in these forces and considerations: searching for economic security or prestige, having a regular, dependable way of life; having and raising children; escaping from whatever one views as restraining, such as home, parents, school, etc.; and seeking companionship. Whatever the reason, most young adults are married or plan someday to be married. Since any interpersonal relationship is constantly fluctuating, the added stress of a potentially fatal illness can cause it to either flounder or flourish.

Treatment for Hodgkin's disease most frequently is given at a large medical center, necessitating separation from the partner and the establishment of different communication patterns. Telephone calls and weekend visits supplant the day-to-day spontaneous dialogue. The very definite need that the ill partner has for love, attention, and reassurance can facilitate the relationship and give it added meaning. The danger is that the fear, anger, and resentment that either or both might have may interfere with this opportunity for saying how much they need each other during this stressful period.

Parenthood is the third major drama of adulthood. It is a constantly changing situation. Development of the parents is as inevitable as development of the offspring. When a new family is established, considerable investment of energy is directed toward the kind of child-rearing one wishes to carry out. Radiotherapy at a distance from home means separation from children, and the patient who is at home may not feel well enough to participate in activities related to the children. Children can exhibit marked behavior changes due to their shift of emphasis to the ill parent. For example, one school-age son of a 25-year-old factory worker feared that his father would die while in the hospital for a routine staging work-up for stage II disease. This boy found the home environment so uncomfortable that he needed to move out and stay with relatives for several weeks. In addition, the ability to have children may be threatened, depending on the site of the disease and the need for irradiation to the pelvic region. This disruption of expectations of parenthood sometimes causes severe distress.

An important issue for the person with a diagnosis of Hodgkin's disease revolves around the fact that choices may now be limited. How will the disease or treatment limit the person's work goals? How will it affect the relationships with significant others? Are choices in family planning severely limited or eliminated? These issues need to be recognized, verbalized, and accepted for their meaning to the individual's self-concept and well-being. With time, the patient will work out some kind of compromise if necessary. The nurse can facilitate a successful adaptation if the nurse is able to recognize and deal with such issues.

Preceding the initiation of radiotherapy, the patient with Hodgkin's disease has undergone the appropriate diagnostic work-up, which includes a careful history, physical examination, chest x-ray film, lymphangiography, laboratory tests, bone marrow biopsy, and a staging laparotomy unless stage 4 disease is apparent. Frequently treatment is started approximately 2 weeks after laparotomy, so that the patient may still be somewhat weak, anorexic, and uncomfortable with abdominal sutures still in place. Because of the extensive work-up, the patient has had several trying weeks of tests and surgery. This has also been a time when the nursing and medical staff have influenced and informed the patient in varying degrees according to the individual's desire to know and understand the ramifications of the illness. Some patients have asked detailed questions and are able to describe exactly where disease has and has not been found. Others may still be quite overwhelmed with their transition from a "well" person who happened to notice a lump to one who feels worn out and miserable with postoperative discomforts. Perhaps the information given to the patient has not penetrated, or perhaps there has been no desire to question or hear the answers. Many adolescents and young adults have found themselves depending heavily on parents. The recently gained desire for independence often reverts to a strong desire to be taken care of and protected by mother or someone else during this period of stress. One might hypothesize that all patients have this need, and depending on age, personality, social position, and parental availability, varying degrees of expression are allowed. Recognizing the opportunity, the nurse on the unit may be able to meet some of these mothering needs while still fostering adult expression of feelings and providing support for maintaining independence.

When patients are referred to the radiotherapy department, a careful assessment is made of what they have been told, what they have heard and understand, and what they want to know. Almost uniformly patients come to the department with a general feeling of uncertainty, not knowing what is going to happen or why treatments are done in such a manner.

Radiation, unlike surgery, has been poorly understood and accepted for its value in curative cancer treatment. Its use has flourished since the advent of high-energy radiation sources and the development of therapeutic radiology as a separate medical specialty, particularly over the past 20 years. Radiotherapy is still rather mysterious to most nurses and definitely to most patients. For a detailed discussion of radiation therapy, see Chapter 7.

Radiosensitivity is defined as the susceptibility of the cell to lethal injury by ionizing radiation.[5] Cells of the lymphatic system, bone marrow and blood, gastrointestinal epithelium, and gonads are highly radiosensitive. Cells of the skin, salivary glands, kidney, liver, lung, and growing bone and cartilage are moderately radiosensitive. Cells of the nervous system and heart are slightly radiosensitive.[3] Muscle, mature bone, cartilage, and connective tissue are radioresistant. Understanding which types of cells are most easily affected assists in predicting the side effects expected during radiotherapy.

Radiosensitivity is a part of a broader concept of radiovulnerability. Some tissues and resultant tumors have greater radiovulnerability than others.[5] This difference in radiovulnerability between tumor and adjacent normal tissues is termed the therapeutic ratio.[5] All radiotherapeutic techniques must exploit this differential. For example, the practice of fractionating the radiotherapy dose over many days is based on the differences in recovery rate between tumor cells and cells of adjacent structures. Since tumor cells may be less able to repair themselves, they may be more vulnerable to destruction, enhancing the therapeutic ratio. In organized body tissues and systems, repair and generation can also determine the effectiveness of radiation therapy. In the treatment of some tumors there is a narrow margin between vulnerability in the tumor and that of the normal structures. Fortunately, regeneration of the normal cells is accomplished through the ability of surrounding surviving cells to replace those which were destroyed.[5] This is observed in the healing of a moist skin reaction from the periphery and islands of undamaged epithelium. Repair is the replacement of destroyed tissue by some other tissue, such as scar tissue.[5] The size of the treated volume and the anatomic site, as well as the total dose, help determine the long-term function and comfort after regeneration and repair resulting from radiation treatment. For example, minimal scar tissue formation in apices of the lungs will not hinder the respiratory function of the individual who received mantle irradiation, whereas a larger volume of lung tissue injury could lead to a compromised respiratory status. Long-term injury and, consequently, compromised function in the organs exposed to the radiation is possible, though the risk is minimal at the usual recommended doses. Such possible late reactions after treatment for Hodgkin's disease include pneumonitis, pericarditis, transverse myelitis, artificial menopause, and impotence, depending on the site of irradiation and other dose-related circumstances.

The development of the megavoltage era in radiotherapy marked the beginning of extended field radiotherapy for Hodgkin's disease. Preceding this era, patients were treated with small fields encompassing the area of gross disease only. Recurrences often were found outside of these fields, necessitating additional treatment, often in close proximity to previously irradiated areas. If this process continued with successive recurrences, treatment that overlapped areas of exposure could lead to irreversible injury of normal tissue and complications. Doses were also more severely limited with kilovoltage radiation because of severe skin reactions and recurrences in the previous fields. Retreatment was then not possible.

Radioactive cobalt (^{60}Co) teletherapy units which emit gamma rays with an energy of approximately 1.25 million electron volts (Mev), and x-ray sources, primarily linear accelerators in the 4 to 8 Mev range, have been used most extensively to deliver the treatments since their introduction in the 1950s. Either type of unit is used equally well as long as there is a treatment distance capability sufficiently great to allow large-field irradiation. Megavoltage, or "supervoltage," radiation, in contrast to the earlier kilovoltage radiation, has the advantage of being more penetrating as well as sparing the surface skin layer from excessively high doses relative to doses at depth. Megavoltage radiation also has better-defined, sharper beam edges and is less injurious to bone tissue than kilovoltage energy levels. Therefore, adequate tumoricidal doses can now be given to the lymph node chains without the severe normal tissue injury seen in earlier years. Doses that are currently being recommended are in the range of 3500 rads in 3½ weeks to 4400 rads in 4 weeks, given in the standard five treatments per week, Monday through Friday.[7] Large fields have the advantage of adequately covering all lymph node areas involved in the disease or at risk without the need for matching boundaries. Gaps leading to underdosed areas or overlaps leading to overdosed areas are the occasional results of trying to match boundaries of adjacent fields.

There are specific indications for using any particular combination of radiation fields and chemotherapy. Factors deciding which particular therapy is given include the patient's age, clinical stage, histopathologic type, and coexistent illness.[7] It would not be appropriate to attempt even a superficial discussion of recommended treatment plans. Briefly, however, to understand patient reactions to radiotherapy, commonly used fields and what they encompass can be outlined as follows[7]:

1. Mantle—includes mediastinal, hilar, and bilateral supraclavicular, infraclavicular, cervical, and axillary node chains, with lead shields shaped to
lungs, heart, and humeral head to block these areas from the direct beam
2. Inverted Y—includes splenic hilar, periaortic, iliac, inguinal, and femoral
node chains, with lead shields to block the rectum and bladder, iliac and
upper femoral bone marrow, and "gap" at junction with mantle field

Other fields, such as the spade field (encompasses the splenic hilar, periaortic,
and common iliac node chains), the periaortic/hepatic field, the periaortic strip
field, the pelvic field, the "Waldeyer" field (encompassing preauricular nodes and
lymphatic tissues of Waldeyer's ring), and the minimantle are reductions, modifica-
tions, or small area additions to the above large fields.

The mantle field extends from the mandible to the diaphragm. Therefore,
normal structures that are being exposed to the radiation and are thus affected
include the lower salivary glands and taste buds, throat, esophagus, bone marrow,
skin, and small portions of the lungs. The inverted-Y field extends from the diaphragm to the lower border of the pelvis. Blocking, as described above, eliminates
significant exposure to the bladder, rectum, and some of the intestine, but portions of the stomach, intestines, and bone marrow are included. This, in general,
describes those areas that are typically treated.

No sooner has the patient begun to realize the diagnosis when questions arise
as to what the treatment will be. To some people the concept of a slow, invisible
process of destroying the disease is less acceptable than the sharp, quick use of
the knife to excise. For many patients the only visible disease was removed with
the diagnostic biopsy, and this is reassuring. For others, doubt melts away only
as examining fingers can document the reduction of a mass. The acute reactions,
frequently termed side effects, are what concerns the patient and the nurse during
a course of radiotherapy.

One can conclude from the discussion of radiosensitivity that certain tissues
included within the typical mantle or inverted-Y treatment fields will evidence
more injury and consequent side effects than others because of varying radio-
sensitivities. Side effects during radiotherapy depend on the site of treatment, except for the complex of symptoms, often termed "radiation sickness," that include lassitude, fatigue, and nausea and vomiting. The cause is not defined, and
there are great individual differences.

Patients are prepared for what they can expect during treatment. All questions
about equipment and the reasons for certain positions and techniques are answered,
and pamphlets describing radiotherapy are shared. There is great need for confidence. Patients who feel that the physician or those working with them have be-
trayed them, misled them, or allowed them to be unduly injured have another
emotional problem superimposed on that incurred by the disease. Therefore, patients receiving upper mantle irradiation are informed that they will experience
some degree of dry mouth, loss of taste, swallowing discomfort, skin redness and
dry peeling in the treatment fields, loss of hair at the back of the neck and under

the arms, reduction of white blood count, and possibly tiredness, nausea, and vomiting.

Patients receiving periaortic strip irradiation usually have minimal side effects consisting of mild fatigue and nausea. Patients receiving an inverted-Y field are informed that they may experience some tiredness, nausea and vomiting, diarrhea, white blood count depression, and skin dryness and redness with peeling, most likely in the groin area. Radiation injury to the gonads is also discussed. In male patients transient aspermia occurs, but recovery of spermatogenesis has been documented by the natural fatherhood of some men irradiated several years previously.[7] In female patients, ovarian function is usually permanently abolished by doses of over 500 to 800 rads absorbed by both ovaries. Oophoropexy (moving the ovaries, pedicles, and tubes midline and securing them to the uterus) and lead blocking shaped to protect the midsagittal point have spared many women of this loss. Kaplan[7] states that more than 60% of the young female patients receiving these precautions have continued or have later resumed normal menstrual function. Patients need to be informed of this option prior to laparotomy so that the oophoropexy can be easily accomplished at the time of surgery.

The effects of radiotherapy are primarily in four main areas: (1) nutritional status, (2) appearance and activity, (3) hematologic status, and (4) life goals and satisfaction.

Factors that affect nutritional status are many. The patient receiving upper mantle irradiation usually experiences a dry mouth, since the submandibular salivary gland function is altered early, often by the beginning of the second week of therapy. Additional fluid with meals is necessary. Some patients find that a mixture of half glycerine and half mouthwash in a pleasant flavor adds some temporary relief throughout the day. An esophagitis reported as "it hurts when I swallow" usually occurs during the second or third week. In a small study that I conducted, it was found that of 12 patients receiving irradiation to the neck and mediastinum for Hodgkin's disease, 6 patients, or 50%, reported esophagitis for the first time on either day 13 or day 15 after the initiation of treatment. Soft foods, without pepper or excessive spices, at mild temperature, neither very hot nor very cold, are the most tolerable. Aspirin gum, if not used to the point of gastric irritation, eases sore throat pain for some individuals. Various anesthetic lozenges are soothing for some patients. For those patients who experience significant discomfort and consequently decrease oral intake, pain medications are also prescribed to take before eating.

Loss of taste or taste distortion occurs due to the radiation effect on the taste buds. Loss of taste was reported by 73% of patients in the small study sample and began primarily between days 13 and 22. It leaves the person with little incentive to eat. The nurse's understanding, encouragement, and ideas for highly nutritious, palatable foods that the patient can try may help to maintain the patient's intake during this period.

The discomfort and difficulty with eating are not minor problems, especially when combined with nausea. For the patient who came to therapy feeling well, the symptoms radiation produces, though expected, represent the reality of the illness. Symptomatic treatment has varying levels of success, sometimes leaving the patient still feeling rather miserable. The effect these symptoms have on the patient's attitude and nutritional status is significant. The distinction between "tolerated therapy well" and "tolerated therapy poorly" lies not so much in the number or severity of symptoms experienced but in how the patient dealt with them. For example, one young man, tense and silent, exerted little effort to follow recommendations for alleviating his sore throat pain and persisted in repeatedly spitting out the thick saliva and declining to take in adequate palatable nourishment. He lost 22 pounds during therapy and consequently felt and looked debilitated. In contrast, another gentleman, who was able to say, "Okay, this isn't easy, but I want to do well," tried various ways of making himself feel better in order to be able to eat enough to maintain his weight. The nurse must be careful to avoid becoming insensitive to the differences in each person's experience of radiotherapy. It is of some reassurance to tell the patient that the symptoms are usual and expected, and that they will subside gradually after treatment is completed. It is easy to superficially leave it at that, but this limits the patient's need to share his own specific sensations and concerns. The nurse who looks at each patient as different is better able to plan how the patient can live with the side effects.

Anorexia is one symptom for which there is no pill, and the patient may either conquer it or be conquered by it. People who matter to the patient, whether they be family, friends, or professionals, can influence the patient to put the extra effort into eating, even though there is no appetite.

Nausea, which is often a significant component to anorexia is treated symptomatically with antiemetics. Patients frequently need assistance in scheduling these medications most effectively to cover the peak time of nausea. Some patients report feeling worse after taking the medication, and when the nausea is transient and mild, they feel better without the side effects of the pills. The incidence of this symptom is highly variable. Of 10 patients who were monitored while receiving mantle irradiation, 5 reported nausea on at least 2 days. Four of the 5 patients receiving inverted-Y–field irradiation reported nausea during the first and second weeks of treatment. Vomiting is less common, with about 60% of the patients having nausea also experiencing vomiting. The practice of reducing the daily dose until significant nausea and vomiting subside is necessary to ensure tolerance. Diarrhea, if persistent, is treated with medication. The avoidance of foods that particularly irritate the patient's bowels is also recommended.

Appearance and activity are affected by radiotherapy. The marking solution used to delineate the fields is used sparingly in the neck area, since it is not usually covered by clothing. Patients develop a sunburned look in the neck and axillary area near the end of treatment, which, together with loss of hair on the back of the head, changes the patient's appearance. Sensitivity to the patient's perception of these changes is important, and measures to help the patient feel neat and attractive aid in reducing their impact.

The skin reaction is usually limited to dry peeling, which occurs at the end of treatment or after it is completed. The use of mineral oil, baby oil, or Aquaphor is recommended only if itchiness is a problem. Patients are cautioned not to put anything on the skin before the daily treatment, thus enhancing absorption of radiation at the skin surface. The best policy is to leave the skin alone—no rubbing, scrubbing, exposure to sun, heat, or cold, or application of solutions or lotions. The axillae and groin, due to doses at the skin level and moistness, evidence more tenderness and peeling. Keeping the area clean and open generally allows the healing to occur rapidly without complication.

Tiredness is often pervasive and leaves the person without energy or ambition. Extra rest and sleep are recommended. Some patients need help in reducing their demands on themselves, whereas others need some encouragement to play down the sick role and find activities to alleviate the boredom that accompanies being away from work, school, or other activities.

As stated earlier, blood cells and bone marrow cells are highly radiosensitive. Treatment occasionally must be interrupted temporarily to allow recovery of the white blood cell count and/or platelet count during wide field radiotherapy. Whenever possible, a 2- to 4-week rest period is given to the patient between the completion of the initial field—which should always be the area of predominant disease, either above or below the diaphragm—and the resumption of treatment to the transdiaphragmatic field. For example, irradiation of the mantle would be followed by a 3-week rest period before starting irradiation of a periaortic strip field. Patients are informed of the frequency of blood tests and the rationale for ordering them. For some patients, bone marrow suppression is marked, and they daily wait for the news on their white blood cell count and whether or not they will receive a treatment. Many ideas, relating to nutrition and exercise, on how to stimulate bone marrow production are often tried by the patient, but success is very unpredictable, and investigation into possible methods of stimulating the bone marrow to produce blood cells is needed.

Further research is needed in all the area of patient reactions. The factors that contribute to the differences in patient tolerance to treatment are many, but by studying large groups of patients, one may be able to decipher the relative importance of nutritional status, stage of disease, personality factors, age, etc. High-risk groups of patients might emerge and deserve extra attention. Nausea and vomiting can be quite distressful to the patient, and as yet pharmaceutic treatment is sometimes ineffective. Additional methods of assisting the patient may lie in the realm of the psychologic, as indicated by the wide acceptance recently given to the close interrelationship between the mind and body. Nurses have the obligation in the radiotherapy treatment situation to learn as much as possible about patient reactions. With that knowledge comes a greater opportunity to expand the repertoire of assistance.

The nurse's effectiveness in helping a patient deal with the stresses imposed by radiotherapy depends partly on availability to the patient on a day-to-day basis in the treatment areas. In most radiotherapy departments, the team dealing with the patient consists of the nurse, the physician, and the technician. The technician's primary thrust is the accurate, efficient delivery of the prescribed dose to the precise fields established by the physician. The technician has daily, brief contact with the patient but little opportunity for follow-through on patient problems. The physician's thrust is a careful assessment of the extent of disease, establishment of the appropriate therapy plan, and institution of that plan. The majority of time is spent with new consultations and initiation of new therapies.

The nurse's primary contribution is in daily access to the patient during treatment. The nurse focuses on what effect the diagnosis and treatment are having on the patient's life situation. How have work and family been affected? Are there financial, travel, or other health problems which the nurse could help the patient solve by contacting appropriate agencies? Teaching the patient and family about radiation and its effects and clarifying misconceptions may ease tension and help them to feel more in control. There is no doubt that patients receiving wide-field radiotherapy need a lot of understanding and reassurance as they deal with the side effects of treatment. Since no one approach to nausea, sore throat, or dry mouth is helpful to all patients, the nurse can explore possibilities and aid the patient in adapting to the temporary discomfort most successfully. The nurse can also catch problems early if unusual symptoms arise and can suggest and arrange preliminary screening tests such a x-ray films, cultures, or blood work to enable the physician to better evaluate the problem.

Close communication with the technician and physician is important to keep up-to-date on the medical plan, as well as to successfully interpret information and answer questions regarding the plan and progress of treatment. Basic knowledge of the principles and techniques of radiotherapy is vital to the nurse's ability to be helpful in answering the patient's questions.

Almost as important as technical knowledge is the nurse's skill in interpersonal relationships. The patient needs to feel almost immediately at ease in an atmosphere of openness and acceptance that allows disclosure of whatever is on the patient's mind. Professional helpers, according to Combs and associates,[6] must be thinking, problem-solving people, and the primary tool with which they work is themselves. Using oneself therapeutically takes time, just as sharing and exploring feelings take time. The relationship, which involves an exchange from both parties, is used to say to the patient, "I think you are important," and "I am not afraid of your fear." Being able to face the psychic pain while supported by the helping person aids in clarifying feelings and expressing them, which eases the disquiet they cause. The relationship established during the weeks of radiotherapy, if maintained on follow-up visits, can provide the patient with the continuity so needed and often lacking in large medical centers where patients with Hodgkin's disease are primarily treated. The distinct advantage of nurse involvement in the patient's adaptation to the short- and long-range implications of Hodgkin's disease is yet being defined and established. The rewards to the nurse who commits the time and skill necessary to this endeavor are immeasurable.

REFERENCES

1. American Cancer Society: 74 cancer facts and figures, New York, 1974.
2. Baldy, C.: The lymphomas: Concepts and Current Therapies, Nursing Clinics of North America **7:**763, Dec., 1972.
3. Berdjis, C., editor: Pathology of irradiation, Baltimore, 1971, The Williams & Wilkins Co.
4. Bolin, R. H., and Auld, M. E.: Hodgkin's disease, American Journal of Nursing **74:**1982, Nov., 1974.
5. Buschke, F., and Parker, R. G.: Radiation therapy in cancer management, New York, 1972, Gune & Stratton, Inc.
6. Combs, A. W., Avila, D. L., and Purkey, W. W.: Helping relationships: basic concepts for the helping professions, Boston, 1971, Allyn & Bacon, Inc.
7. Kaplan, H. S.: Hodgkin's disease, Cambridge, Mass., 1972, Harvard University Press.
8. Keller, A. R., Kaplan, H. W., Lukes, R. J., and Rappaport, H.: Correlation of histopathology with other prognostic indicators in Hodgkin's disease, Cancer **22:** 488, Sept., 1968.
9. Perlman, H. H.: Persona: social role and personality, Chicago, 1968, The University of Chicago Press.
10. Schwartz, E. E., editor: The biological basis of radiation therapy, Philadelphia, 1966, J. B. Lippincott Co.

9 Acute lymphocytic leukemia of childhood

care of the child and family

MARGARET LAWLEY MORSE

Before any treatment was available, the mean period of survival for children with acute lymphocytic leukemia was 3 months. In 1948, Dr. Sidney Farber introduced the first effective chemotherapeutic agent, aminopterin, a folic acid antagonist, and reported successful temporary remissions.[17] The length of these temporary remissions gradually increased with the discovery of additional chemotherapeutic agents.

The fact that many children have maintained a continual remission for several years after therapy has been discontinued has led some investigators to consider the disease curable.[23] Many sources, however, indicate that it is premature to speak in terms of cure and more appropriate to consider these children to simply be in long-term remission.

Acute lymphocytic leukemia, in many respects, is no longer an acute disease but a chronic one that often can be controlled to provide many symptom-free years. The increase in the length of survival has accentuated many problems that previously seemed insignificant,[23] including all the problems related to the anxiety of living with the threat of a terminal illness, as well as the many problems related to complications of aggressive therapy. This chapter will describe current therapies that have led to the striking increase in the length of survival. Emphasis will be placed on the essential nursing contributions to the care of these children and their families.

For discussion of background information on pathophysiology, etiology, incidence prognosis, and signs and symptoms, see Weetman and Baehner.[26]

INDUCTION OF REMISSION
Medical management at time of admission

A child who is admitted with suspected acute lymphocytic leukemia should be examined carefully with special reference to any signs of infection, severe anemia, or bleeding. Necessary laboratory studies include a complete blood count, platelet count, coagulation studies, kidney and liver functions, and cultures as indicated. A bone marrow examination must be done to verify the diagnosis and to distinguish between the various types of leukemia. A lumbar puncture is necessary to determine whether central nervous system disease is present.

Once the diagnosis is established, several preparatory and supportive measures are instituted before chemotherapy can be started. Packed cells, platelet transfusions, and antibiotics should be given as indicated. Another concern in beginning therapy for a child with leukema is the control of the hyperuricemia usually present at the time of diagnosis. This condition occurs because of the rapid turnover of purines resulting from the increased cellular proliferation and from the breakdown of leukemic cells.[26] Chemotherapy will cause a further increase in the uric acid levels due to the rapid lysis of leukemic cells, and the uric acid should be at a normal level before any chemotherapy is begun.

To control hyperuricemia, certain precautions are taken routinely. Intravenous fluids are started and continued for the first several days of treatment to assure adequate hydration, and the child is encouraged to increase oral fluid intake. Sodium bicarbonate may be added to the intravenous fluids to alkalize the urine, since uric acid is more soluble in alkaline than in acid urine. The urine pH should be maintained above 7.0. Allopurinol, given orally, blocks the production of uric acid by inhibiting xanthine oxidase, an enzyme that acts as a catalyst in the formation of uric acid from purines. This drug is given to all children with leukemia at the time of diagnosis.

Therapy

The goal of therapy in acute lymphocytic leukemia is the achievement of remission. Remission is determined on bone marrow examination by the presence of normal cellularity and less than 5% blasts. The peripheral blood count must be within normal limits, and the child must be free of symptoms attributed to the disease and have a normal physical examination.[20,26] Most authorities recommend the combination of vincristine and prednisone to induce remission. These agents, when used together, have been shown to be effective in inducing remission in 86% to 91% of children.[15,23] Side effects and nursing implications of administration of the chemotherapeutic agents mentioned are included in the table that appears at the end of the chapter.

Vincristine is given intravenously once each week for approximately 6 weeks. Prednisone is given orally in three divided doses per 24 hours for 6 weeks and then tapered gradually over another week. It should be noted that additional agents such as L-asparaginase may be added to this regimen at certain institutions in an attempt to improve the rate of remission induction.

Role of the nurse

Initial nursing contact. When a child and family first arrive at the hospital, they are very anxious and frightened. They may or may not have been told that the child was being referred because of the suspicion of leukemia, but they do know that something is seriously wrong. They usually have had little time to prepare for the admission. Nuring plays a major role in aiding their adjustment during this crucial period. The most important nursing goals during this initial contact are to establish a helping relationship and to begin to assess the special needs of this family unit. One of the first concerns of most parents is whether or not they may stay with their child. Allowing parents to stay with their seriously ill child and to participate in the care is crucial to the psychologic well-being of both the child and the family.[13] Parents are especially needed to stay with young children. However, in our experience, even the most independent teenager may need to have parents present during the first few days of hospitalization to help in facing the crisis that leukemia presents.

Preparation of the child and family for medical procedures. It is very important to verify the diagnosis as soon as possible to shorten the painful period of uncertainty for the family. Preparation of the child and the family for the many procedures to be completed during the first few hours after admission is an important nursing responsibility. The child will have blood work, a bone marrow, and a spinal tap, and intravenous fluids will be started within a short period of time. The nurse should explain these procedures to the child and the family and promise to stay with the child during this time. For the younger child, simple explanations are best. We have found that using a doll is helpful to show the child the positions to assume and what will be done. Volunteers furnish the hospital with a continual supply of small cloth dolls so that each child may keep one.

After these procedures, the child, with the help of the nurse, may perform "bone marrow procedures" and start "intravenous fluids" on the dolls. It is difficult for a young child to see any benefit from needles, and they are often interpreted as attacks or punishment for some misdeed.[21] The child who is allowed to handle and play with some of the hospital equipment is able to gain better control of a confusing and stressful situation.

Older children need to know what is going to be done and the reason it is necessary. A body diagram is often helpful in describing procedures to older children, since they are interested in the anatomy and physiology involved, such as which bones are used for bone marrow examinations or how the spinal fluid is obtained.[21]

INTERVIEW WITH PARENTS. When the initial blood work and bone marrow examination have been completed and the diagnosis is established, the physician should arrange for a conference with the child's parents. It should take place with both parents present in a quiet private setting away from the child's room. At this first interview the physician from the hematology-oncology staff, the house officer responsible for the child's care, and the nurse who will be working with the child and the family should be present. The presence of these staff members enables the parents to begin to form an early and confident relationship with the individuals caring for their child.[1]

The primary purpose of the initial conference is to inform the parents of the diagnosis in a direct but sympathetic manner. The parents should be allowed to express their fears and concerns. Their reaction and ability to comprehend further information should set the tone of the interview. Several aspects of the disease need to be discussed with the parents during the initial hospitalization. How much is covered at the first interview will vary according to the individual needs of the parents.

It is helpful to question the parents to determine their knowledge of leukemia so that a firmer basis for future discussions can be developed. Parents need to know that the cause of leukemia is unknown and that it did not occur because of something they did or did not do. They should be reassured that leukemia is not hereditary and that it is extremely unlikely that their other children will develop the disease. The goals of treatment and the concept of remission should be discussed in a general manner. Parents are encouraged that the chances of obtaining remission are good and that the child will feel well during remission. They are told that the length of remission varies from several months to several years, and that it is impossible to predict how well their own child will respond to therapy. However, if the child has many of the poor prognostic signs (black children, children under 1 year or over 10 years of age, a high initial white blood count [over 20,000], hepatosplenomegaly, and massive adenopathy, especially mediastinal[5,17,26]), parents are usually informed of this fact.

Parents need to be assured that the therapy their child will receive is the best available. The concept of cooperative research through national group efforts is explained to let the family know that physicians all over the country caring for children with leukemia are in constant communication with one another. It is also helpful to stress to the parents that a discovery made anywhere in the world is quickly communicated to others involved in the care of these children.[9]

The final area that needs to be discussed at the first conference concerns the content and extent of information to be given to the child and the siblings. The age of the child, the wishes of the parents, and the philosophy of those caring for the child are the determining factors. In our experience we have found it to be unrealistic and unwise to keep the diagnosis from the child. Children are becoming increasingly more aware of leukemia and its treatment through health classes and television programs. Many of the older children have guessed the diagnosis before it is confirmed. By the time children return to school, many of their classmates will have heard the diagnosis and may ask questions concerning it.

Several years ago the child guidance clinic at our hospital conducted a program of group sessions for adolescents with possible terminal illnesses. The group consisted of approximately 10 children with leukemia or other malignancies. Only 3 children had been told of their diagnosis directly. The others had never been told, and their parents firmly believed that they had no idea of the seriousness of their condition. During the second group session the children began discussing their diagnoses. They went around the table, and each child stated his diagnosis and what he understood about it. All the children but one knew exactly what was wrong with them and how they were progressing. Many had been to the library and read extensively about their illness. These children also recognized that their parents did not want them to know their diagnoses and therefore had never discussed their fears or concerns with anyone. Children who are aware of the diagnosis but also realize that their parents do not want them to know become lonely and isolated. They attempt to protect their parents as the parents attempt to shield their child.[2]

The initial reaction of most parents is that they do not want their child told of the diagnosis because they wish to provide protection from this painful experience. We do not instruct parents but listen and talk with them. The majority of parents will soon realize that telling their child the diagnosis in a sensitive manner is much less frightening than having the child find out in another way. Siblings should be informed of the diagnosis in the same way. Since acute lymphocytic leukemia can now be viewed as a chronic illness that can last for years, the child may literally grow up with the disease. We need to approach it as such. If a child has diabetes or cystic fibrosis, no one would suggest that we not inform the child of the nature of the illness. It now seems appropriate that we approach leukemia in much the same way, realizing that the child may live with the disease and its therapies for many years.

TALKING WITH THE CHILD. The exact content of the discussion with the child varies according to age and the questions asked. The preschool child is primarily concerned with day-to-day happenings, how many shots there will be, when the return home will occur, and, most important, whether the parents may stay at the hospital. A simple explanation of the reasons for all the tests and medicine is necessary. It is helpful to relate the explanation to something the child can see, such as "the medicines will help make the bruises go away."

The preschool child often experiences much guilt concerning the illness, believing that he caused it in some way.[21] Fred, a 5-year-old boy referred for treatment after amputation of his left arm for a malignant tumor, had been told that he had cancer. When asked what he thought had caused it, he said: "I smoked once. My brother gave me a cigarette, and I smoked it. The smoke went in here (pointed to his mouth) and then went to my arm, and that gave me cancer." It is important to find out what thoughts the child may have and to give reassurance that nothing the child did had caused the illness.

The discussion for the school-age child or teenager is individualized depending on the child's maturity. In general, the child is given the diagnosis of leukemia and is asked to relate any information they had been told. Leukemia is then explained in basic terms, and the child is told that although there is no cure, there are medicines that can control it. The concept of remission is explained, and the child is encouraged to ask questions. Often the child is overwhelmed and will not ask anything at this time. The physician and nurse should let the child know that they will be seeing him frequently and will be available for questions as they arise.

Other staff members, such as the occupational therapist and child life worker, can be helpful to the child in the hospital. Continuation of normal childhood activities provides the child with an important psychologic outlet. Our hospital also has a school program, and the child is encouraged to attend class and keep up on assignments while in the hospital. If possible, the child should return to school soon after being discharged from the hospital.

POINTS OF GUIDANCE. The diagnosis of leukemia is difficult for parents to accept. They cannot believe that their beautiful child, who has always been so healthy, is suddenly seriously ill. One of the best ways a nurse can help parents at this stage is to simply allow them to express their anger and fears.

The full impact of the diagnosis develops gradually. A young mother whose 5-year-old daughter was newly diagnosed with leukemia told many of the other parents that her little girl just had a "light case" of leukemia. The diagnosis and its implications had been explained fully, but the mother was indicating that she could only accept its impact gradually.

Early guidance will often help the family to become aware of common problems and enable them to deal with them more effectively. Overindulgence and overprotection occur frequently. We encourage parents to try to treat the leukemia child as normally as possible. Parents need to know that their child will feel safer and happier when limits and expectations are the same as before the illness.[3] Realistically it may not be possible for parents to treat their child as if nothing had happened, but with a more knowledgeable approach they may at least attempt to do so.

The social worker is an important member of the care team and should interview families during the first admission. This enables the parents to express many of their feelings and facilitates their adjustment during this stressful time. The social worker can also evaluate the family's financial situation and refer them for appropriate aid. Depending on the assessment of the family's needs, the social worker may see them continually or at intervals as problems arise.

Helping the family feel comfortable with their understanding of the disease and the care their child will require at home is very important. The physician will outline the treatment plan and discuss side effects of the medications during the first few days of hospitalization; the nurse should follow up by talking to the child's parents daily, providing clarification, review, or additional information as needed. Verbal discussions are more meaningful when accompanied by written information that can be referred to at a later date. Pamphlets such as *Childhood Leukemia: a pamphlet for Parents*[11] contain much helpful information. Common side effects of chemotherapy are also discussed and written on a small card that the parents may keep for reference. Side effects of the drugs are presented in terms of symptoms that the child may display. The older child or teenager also needs to know the common side effects so as not to be frightened if they occur.

Of all the side effects, the ones that affect the child's appearance are usually the most difficult for the child and the family. Weight gain from prednisone and alopecia from vincristine and/or later radiation are very distressing. The child needs to understand that these changes will occur but that they will be temporary. We recommend that the child and the parents begin looking for a wig before any hair loss occurs so that a wig may be chosen that closely resembles the child's natural hair color and style.

Other points to be discussed with parents include specific drugs and vaccines to be avoided. We ask parents to refrain from giving their child vitamins that contain folic acid, since they may interfere with the action of methotrexate, which the child will receive for maintenance. Children with leukemia should not take aspirin because of its effects on platelet function.[20] Due to the immunosuppression caused by the basic disease and chemotherapy, children with leukemia should never receive live virus vaccines.[26] We ask parents to notify us if the child is exposed to any communicable disease. Chickenpox, especially, can be serious for the child with leukemia, and steps should be taken to prevent its development after exposure.

Many of the parents' questions and concerns cannot be anticipated during the first admission. We encourage parents to write down their questions after they are home, since often they otherwise will be forgotten during clinic visits. It is extremely important for the parents to have staff members' phone numbers for use if necessary. We encourage parents to call if they are concerned about anything. We also tell them that their local physician will be notified when the child is discharged and may also be consulted.

Central nervous system prophylaxis

Therapy. The central nervous system often serves as a reservoir for leukemic cells. It has been shown that systemic chemotherapy does not penetrate this area in effective concentration and therefore does not eradicate leukemic cells. This has been attributed to the failure of antileukemic drugs to cross the blood-brain barrier.[22] A lumbar puncture is done on all children at the time of diagnosis to check for the presence of leukemic cells. Very few children will have central nervous system disease detectable at diagnosis. However, without specific prophylactic therapy to this area, approximately half of all children with acute lymphocytic leukemia will develop overt central nervous system disease within the first year.[20] Prophylactic therapy has been shown to effectively prevent the development of central nervous system disease in the majority of children. Study VII from St. Jude's Hospital indicated that prophylactic therapy with craniospinal irradiation decreased the development of central nervous system disease from 50% to 4.4%.[23]

Irradiation therapy and intrathecal methotrexate used individually or in combination have been found to be effective prophylactic therapy. The type of therapy used for an individual child will vary according to the philosophy of the physician or institution. The important aspect, however, is that all newly diagnosed children with acute lymphocytic leukemia must receive some form of effective central nervous system prophylaxis.

Role of the nurse. This phase of therapy usually lasts approximately 3 weeks.

Radiotherapy is given Monday through Friday for approximately 2 to 3 weeks, and intrathecal methotrexate is given twice a week for 3 weeks. Therapy may be completed on an outpatient basis if the family lives close enough to the medical center. The child who must be admitted may attend school at the hospital and go home on weekends.

In preparation for radiotherapy, young children need to know that this procedure will not hurt but that they will be in a room by themselves and may be restrained so that they cannot move. Their eyes are also shielded for protection. The reasons that the marks are drawn on the skin should be explained. It is helpful to rehearse the procedures with the child or to demonstrate them by using a doll. Older children are more interested in details such as how radiotherapy works. Many of the parents' questions concerning risks of therapy and the possibilities of latent side effects are best discussed with the radiotherapist.

Increased fatigability, nausea, and vomiting occur as side effects of cranial irradiation, and parents should be told of this possibility. The child and the family have already been prepared for the alopecia that will occur. A mild soap should be used on the area of skin included in the radiation field, but creams and lotions should not be applied to the skin without consulting the radiotherapist. The marks drawn on the skin often rub off slightly, and the child may wish to wear old clothes because the marks sometimes leave a stain. Every precaution should be taken not to remove the lines, however. Irradiation therapy sometimes suppresses the blood count, and a complete blood count should be done at set intervals.

It is difficult for young children to cope with intrathecal methotrexate therapy at such frequent intervals. At least one spinal tap has been done in the past, but additional preparation should be given, since some children may not remember what was done or what was expected of them. During this phase of frequent taps, young children may especially benefit from hospital play, such as bringing a doll that also "receives a spinal tap."

MAINTENANCE
Therapy

After prophylactic treatment to the central nervous system has been completed, therapy is initiated to maintain the remission. The two drugs that are most effective in maintaining remission are methotrexate and 6-mercaptopurine.[23] Currently most treatment protocols include a combination of these two agents. Some regimens may also add cyclophosphamide or vincristine and prednisone "pulses" at set intervals.[23]

The rationale for using a combination of drugs for maintenance is that it is advantageous to attack the leukemic cells in a variety of ways simultaneously.[14] Protocols are designed to offer the maximum leukemic cell kill with as little increase in toxicity as possible.[26] It is not practical to list the exact combinations or timing of administration of these drugs because these will vary depending on the preferences of the individual physician or institution. Drug regimens also change frequently as results of current studies indicate areas of improvement.

Complications during remission

Nonbacterial infections. The combination of more aggressive drug and irradiation therapy has led to increased survival for children with acute lymphocytic leukemia. However, this intensive therapy is also responsible for the increased susceptibility of these children to nonbacterial infections. Organisms include *Pneumocystis carinii,* fungi such as *Candida albicans* and *Aspergillus fumigatus,* and viruses such as varicella-zoster and cytomegalovirus.[24]

In our experience, *P. carinii* has caused one of the major life-threatening infections of children in remission. Only 48% to 68% of patients with documented *P. carinii* survive, even with pentamidine isethionate therapy. Although the disease is devastating, it is fortunately an uncommon complication of leukemic therapy.

Viral infections such as varicella and herpes zoster are also of great concern in children with leukemia. We ask parents to notify us immediately of any exposure to chickenpox. If the child is exposed to varicella by someone with whom there has been extended contact, such as a sibling, zoster immune globulin (ZIG) should be given to prevent clinical manifestations of the disease. If a child does develop disseminated varicella or herpes zoster infection, however, it can be life-threatening. These infections may include a varicella pneumonia as well as widespread skin eruptions. Cytosine arabinoside has been found to be helpful in the treatment of disseminated varicella or herpes zoster infections. It is not always effective, however, and further study is needed concerning its use.[18]

Drug toxicities. Methotrexate and 6-mercaptopurine are the best drugs to maintain remission and are included in nearly all maintenance regimens. These drugs are well tolerated, and side effects and toxicities such as marrow suppression can usually be easily controlled through dosage adjustments. An important side effect of methotrexate therapy is the development of gastrointestinal ulcerations. These lesions usually begin in the mouth and may progress down the entire gastrointestinal tract if therapy is continued. It is important to alert the child and the parents that methotrexate should be withheld if mouth ulcers are present.[20]

Another more serious side effect of these drugs is hepatic toxicity. Liver function studies should be obtained every 3 or 4 months during maintenance. If hepatic toxicity occurs, the drugs must be discontinued.[20] Sometimes they may be reinstated when the drug-induced hepatitis is cleared, but often the child can never tolerate them again.

Cessation of therapy

When a child has responded very well to therapy and has remained in continuous bone marrow remission, the question arises as to how long therapy should be continued. In addition to the complication of the chemotherapeutic agents previously described, there is also evidence that prolonged therapy with these drugs may result in permanent damage to the liver or other organs, sterility, and even an increased risk of a second neoplasm. Because of the serious consequences of long-term therapy, these potent drugs should be given only long enough to provide optimal benefits.[23] Many institutions are discontinuing therapy for children who have been in continuous remission for at least 3 years. Currently the rate of relapse of children who have discontinued therapy is being compared to those who have continued therapy.

Role of the nurse. During long periods of remission the child feels physically well, and it is sometimes assumed that there are no problems for either the child or the family. This is not usually true. Living with the threat of a terminal illness creates many sources of stress for the child and the family. The fear of relapse is constantly present. Encouraging open communication between the parents is important in preserving their relationship, and it is also helpful to provide parents with an opportunity to discuss their feelings at the time of a clinic visit. In our clinic the same physician and nurse attempt to see the same children during each visit. In this way they establish a close relationship with the child and the family. The social worker may also see the family during these visits.

Another problem experienced by parents during remission is their tendency to overprotect the child. Although this problem was discussed at the time of diagnosis, it should be explored at subsequent clinic visits. It is not unusual for parents never to leave their child with a babysitter or for the child to be sleeping with the parents. A 6-year-old girl once told me about all of her dolls, which she kept on her bed at home. When I asked her where she found room to sleep, she replied, "Oh, I sleep with mommy; the dolls are my daddy's problem."

At clinic visits, it is important to talk with older children and teenagers concerning their activities. Are they experiencing problems with peers or parents? Often older children and teenagers will bring the problem of overprotection by the parents to the attention of the physician or nurse, and ask for help in convincing the parents to allow a more normal life. One teenage boy with leukemia related that his family and several other families went camping frequently. Usually the parents stayed in a cabin, and the children slept in tents. Since he had been diagnosed as having leukemia, however, he had been made to sleep in the cabin with the adults. Another teenage boy described his situation by saying, "Things are so bad at my house that my grandmother offers me her chair when I walk into the room."

The parents described in the examples were good parents who were trying to do what was best for their child but simply needed some guidance. Parents are often too frightened to change these behaviors immediately, and the counseling should be a very gradual process. During long phases of illness the parents often focus completely on the child instead of relating to one another. If the child dies, there is little left to keep the parents together, and divorce often occurs. Some studies have shown that as many as 50% of marriages end in divorce after the death of a child from leukemia.[16]

Another area that sometimes presents problems for the children is school.

For a detailed discussion on the return of a leukemic child to school, see Chapter 19.

The atmosphere of the clinic is also very important. At our clinic a child life worker plans activities for the children in the waiting room. Such activities as making ice cream, showing movies, or participating in a variety of arts and crafts projects are common. The secretaries, laboratory technicians, and nurses also are involved in the planning of special activities for holidays or special occasions.

RELAPSES

If 50% of the children will remain in continuous first remission for at least 5 years, this means that approximately 50% will relapse before that time. There are three main areas in which relapse may occur: bone marrow, central nervous system, and testes. Other areas such as the ovaries or kidneys may also contain sites of leukemic infiltration but are seldom clinically evident.

Bone marrow

Bone marrow relapses account for the majority of relapses in children with acute lymphocytic leukemia. Symptoms of a bone marrow relapse are similar to those at the time of diagnosis. However, because bone marrow examinations are done at intervals of every 3 or 4 months, a relapse may be discovered in children who are totally asymptomatic.

Bone marrow relapse occurs because the leukemic cells have become resistant to the maintenance chemotherapy. When a child has a bone marrow relapse while on 6-mercaptopurine and methotrexate maintenance, it means that these drugs are no longer effective in controlling the disease. Induction agents such as vincristine and prednisone can often be used repeatedly to induce remissions, although the rate of response decreases with each subsequent induction.[25] Other agents are also known to be effective in producing remission in some children with acute lymphocytic leukemia, including L-asparaginase, cytosine arabinoside, adriamycin, cyclophosphamide, and daunomycin.[6,25]

The choice of chemotherapeutic agents used for reinduction and eventual maintenance therapies will vary depending on drugs previously administered and on the preference of the treating physician. Subsequent remissions are generally of shorter duration than the first. The concept of total therapy includes the most efficient drugs used in combination to hopefully prolong the first remission indefinitely. If a child relapses on the best regimen available, the chances of long-term survival are greatly decreased.

Central nervous system

The incidence of central nervous system relapse has been greatly decreased by the use of prophylactic therapy. However, it still occurs as the initial site of relapse in a small number of children. The most common signs and symptoms of central nervous system leukemic infiltration are related to the increased intracranial pressure that it causes. Common symptoms include nausea, vomiting, lethargy, head-ache, and papilledema. Stiff neck, cranial nerve palsies, and even convulsions may sometimes occur.[22]

The diagnosis of central nervous system leukemia is established by examination of the spinal fluid. The presence of ten or more leukemic cells per cubic milli-meter of spinal fluid is considered diagnostic of central nervous system leukemic involvement.[4] If a child develops central nervous system leukemia after previ-ous prophylactic therapy, the central nervous system relapse is usually treated with an alternate method of treatment than originally given. For example, if a child receives craniospinal irradiation for prophylaxis, intrathecal methotrexate might possibly be given at the time of relapse or vice versa. Methotrexate is also used in children with persistent meningeal leukemia.[22]

Testes

Testicular involvement occurs less frequently than central nervous system re-lapse. It is seldom bilateral and is usually manifested by a painless unilateral testic-ular enlargement. The diagnosis is confirmed by biopsy, and treatment consists of irradiation to the involved gonad.[7]

Role of the nurse

A relapse of any type is extremely stressful for both the child and the family. Many parents relate that it is like "hearing the diagnosis all over again." Often their lives have just returned to normal, and now the child must face the changes in appearance all over again. Sometimes the child has just discarded a wig and must now wear it again.

The physical care and emotional support of the child and the family at the time of bone marrow relapse is similar to the care at diagnosis. The child should be admitted and well hydrated before chemotherapy is begun. Central nervous sys-tem relapse and testicular relapse may require hospitalization for radiation treat-ment if the family lives too far away to drive to the hospital daily.

OTHER TYPES OF THERAPY
Immunotherapy

Immunotherapy in the treatment of acute lymphocytic leukemia is in the early stages of investigation. In 1969 Georges Mathé reported successful remission main-tenance in some patients using BCG vaccine and/or irradiated leukemic cells.[17] Im-munotherapy is based on the concept that once the child is in complete remission, the leukemic cell burden is significantly decreased, and immunotherapy may then be effective in eliminating the last remaining cells. Mathé's results were not substan-tiated however, by a study completed in England or by a study done by Children's Cancer Study Group, which indicated no differences between children receiving BCG and those receiving no therapy. More study is necessary to answer the ques-tion of what role immunotherapy will play in the future treatment of acute lympho-cytic leukemia.[17]

Bone marrow transplants

The goal of bone marrow transplantation in acute lymphocytic leukemia is to completely eliminate the child's leukemic cells by administering high doses of chemotherapy or total body irradiation. Bone marrow cells from an HL-A identical donor, usually a sibling, are then infused into the leukemic child with the hope of repopulating the bone marrow. In general, the results have been very discouraging, and this form of treatment is reserved for children whose disease has become refractory to all other conventional forms of therapy.[25]

TERMINAL PHASE
Causes of death

Infection is the major cause of death in acute lymphocytic leukemia in both remission and relapse and accounts for 70% of all deaths. Bleeding is the second leading cause of death, but the availability of platelet transfusions has reduced the risk of fatal hemorrhage significantly.[19] Although fatal infections during remission are primarily due to nonbacterial agents, infections occurring during periods of relapse are mainly bacterial in origin.[18] Protozoal, viral, and fungal infections also occur.

When the disease no longer responds to any of the effective drugs available for the treatment of acute lymphocytic leukemia, the child is dying. At this point, susceptibility to a variety of infectious agents is due to granulocytopenia. Episodes of bleeding due to his thrombocytopenia may also occur, thus leading to death from one or a combination of these causes.

Meaning of death to the child

Many of the child's fears will be related to the concept of death. The very young child, under 3 years of age, sees himself and his parents as a unit. There is no real awareness of personal death, but there is a sense of the parents' unhappiness and fears that separation is near. The child from 3 to 5 years of age sees himself as a distinct individual and is developing an awareness that people can die. The concept of death depends greatly on the child's life experiences.[8]

The grade-school child usually is developing strong religious beliefs. Dreams about heaven reassure the child that life continues after death. For the young adolescent who is striving to become self-sufficient, illness and eventual death represent an end to valued independence. Rejection by his peers may come at a time when acceptance is needed most. Loneliness and resentment occur because of the realization that death is coming when life, with all that it has to offer, is just beginning. The older adolescent has developed more self-confidence, is less dependent on peers, and has the ability to deeply care for others. This individual now must grieve for the loss of all these meaningful relationships.[8]

Meaning of death to the family

The death of a child is the greatest tragedy most parents will ever face. Many young parents have had little experience with death ever before in their life. To be suddenly faced with the death of their child may be overwhelming. For all parents the death of a child represents the loss of a personal creation, the object of their love and care.[10]

Role of the nurse

What can a nurse do to ease the dying child's fears and help the family cope? The child's hospital room becomes the center of the environment, for the child may never go home again. Nurses have the responsibility to help the child feel safe and comfortable. One way to do so is to make the hospital as much like home as possible. Of course, this means allowing the parents to stay. It also means allowing siblings and best friends to visit. Eight-year-old Martin's greatest wish was to be able to hold his infant twin brother and sister. Even though he was too weak to hold them, his parents laid them next to him in bed, and he was pleased.

For a teenager, making the hospital room seem like home often means bringing the stereo and favorite albums to the hospital. For Joe it meant bringing the carburetor from his motorcycle into his room, even though he seldom felt well enough to work on it and knew that he would probably never ride it again.

The visit of a favorite pet can mean very much to a dying child. Sometimes a child may go to the lobby to see a pet, or if the pet is small, it may be brought to the room. Twelve-year-old David's favorite pet was a guinea pig that was due to deliver at any time. He had calculated the expected delivery date and even certain genetic probabilities such as sex, number, and color of the offspring. Since David's guinea pig was admitted with him, David was able to follow her progress. The babies were delivered on schedule, and all David's probabilities proved to be reliable.

It should be noted that one of the goals of therapy in leukemia is to keep the child out of the hospital as much as possible. If parents care for their dying child at home, they need nursing support through home visits and frequent communication. Many children and their families will feel too anxious and frightened at home and choose to come into the hospital.

Staff members are often worried about what to say to the dying child or afraid of questions that might be asked. In our experience children have seldom asked direct questions about death. Green[12] has described three basic questions that children express verbally or through their behavior: (1) Am I safe? (2) Will there be a trusted person with me so that I won't be alone? and (3) Will you make me feel all right? Since a child communicates more through behavior than through words, more is communicated through our behavior and touch than verbally. Holding a small child on your lap is more comforting than just sitting next to the bed. Holding the dying teenager's hand and giving reassurance that you will be there communicates far more than words alone.

SUMMARY

The care of children with acute lymphocytic leukemia and their families is becoming increasingly complex. Chemotherapy for acute leukemia has been de-

Table 3. Chemotherapeutic agents*

Drug	Route of adminis-tration	Mode of action	Toxic and side effects	Related nursing care
Adriamycin	IV	Believed to retard DNA synthesis; precise mode of action unknown	Oral ulceration, anorexia, gastrointestinal upsets, alopecia and cardiac toxicity; extravasation causes induration	Heart failure after cumulative doses—observe ECG prior to each injection; guard against infiltration
L-Asparaginase	IM	Deprives leukemic cells of L-Asparagine; lympholytic, prevents entry into S-phase	Allergic reactions, fever, nausea and vomiting, impaired liver and kidney function; pancreatitis, diabetes	Observe for allergic reactions; test urine for glucose daily
Cyclophospha-mide	PO IV	Alkylating agent; inhibits DNA synthesis, arrests cells in mitosis, and prevents entry into S-phase	Leukopenia, hemorrhagic cystitis, alopecia, nausea and vomiting	Give early in day; push fluids; Hematest urine; may need antiemetic
Cytosine arabinoside	IV SQ	Pyrimidine antagonist; inhibits DNA synthesis, synchronizes cells in S-phase, and recruits cells from G_0 to G_1	Bone marrow depression, nausea and vomiting, oral ulcerations	May need antiemetic
Daunomycin	IV	Cytocidal; complexes DNA	Bone marrow depression, oral ulcerations, gastrointestinal upsets, phlebitis at injection site; cardiac toxicity	Heart failure after cumulative dose; observe ECG prior to each injection

*Based on data from Nathan, D. G., and Oski, F. A.: Hematology of infancy and childhood, Philadelphia, 1974, W. B. Saunders Co., and Weetman, R. M., and Baehner, R. L.: Management of acute leukemia, Current Problem in Pediatrics **3:**1-52, Aug., 1973.

Table 3. Chemotherapeutic agents—cont'd

Drug	Route of adminis- tration	Mode of action	Toxic and side effects	Related nursing care
6-Mercapto- purine	PO	Purine antag- onist; inhibits DNA and RNA syn- thesis	Bone marrow de- pression, liver toxicity	Allopurinol blocks excretion of 6MP; dosage of 6MP must be reduced by half if patient is tak- ing allopurinol
Methotrexate	PO IV IM	Folic acid an- tagonist; de- prives leu- kemic cell of folic acid and therefore inhibits DNA synthe- sis, synchro- nizes cells in S-phase	Bone marrow de- pression, liver toxicity, oral and gastrointes- tinal ulcerations	Withhold medica- tion and notify physician if mouth ulcers present
Prednisone	PO	Lympholytic agent, pre- vents entry into S-phase	Cushingoid mani- festations, osteo- porosis, hyper- tension	Give drug with meals or snack to prevent gas- trointestinal irri- tation; monitor blood pressure; restrict salty foods
Vincristine	IV	Inhibits flow of cells from G_0 to G_1, arrests cells in mitosis	Neurotoxicity (jaw pain, pares- thesia, loss of deep tendon re- flexes, constipa- tion), alopecia; injection site ex- travasation causes indura- tion	Guard against any infiltration dur- ing administra- tion
Pentamidine isethionate (not a che- mothera- peutic agent, used to treat *Pneumo- cystis carinii* pneumonia)	IM	Protozoacidal agent	Pain at injection site, sterile ab- scess formation, hypoglycemia after 5 to 7 days of treatment	Monitor blood glucose levels

scribed as being "as highly developed a specialty as cardiac surgery."[15] Similarly, providing quality comprehensive nursing care for these children and their families requires very specialized nursing skills.

One of the ways in which nursing is meeting this challenge is through the development of a variety of expanded nursing roles. The clinical nursing specialist in pediatrics or child psychiatry, the nurse clinician, or the pediatric nurse associate may be involved in the care of these children and their families. Overall, providing quality care for these children requires a well-coordinated interdisciplinary team approach. This team includes all the medical professionals at the hospital or clinic, as well as various resource persons within the community setting.

Acute lymphocytic leukemia of childhood may no longer be considered an inevitably fatal disease. As therapy improves and survival is extended, the long-term psychologic as well as medical needs of these children become increasingly apparent. Caring for these children and their families through all phases of treatment is one of the most rewarding roles in all of nursing.

REFERENCES

1. Ablin, A. R., and others: A conference with the family of a leukemic child, American Journal of Diseases of Children **122:**362-364, Oct., 1971.
2. Binger, C. M., and others: Childhood leukemia, emotional impact on patient and family, New England Journal of Medicine **280:**414-418, Feb., 20, 1969.
3. Bright, F., and France, Sr. M. L.: The nurse and the terminally ill child, Nursing Outlook **15:**39-42, Sept., 1967.
4. Children's Cancer Study Group Protocol 101, unpublished, 1971.*
5. Children's Cancer Study Group Protocol 141, unpublished, 1974.*
6. Children's Cancer Study Group Protocol 142, unpublished, 1974.*
7. Cornet, J. M.: Acute leukemia, In Barnett, J. L., and Einhorn, A. H., editors: Pediatrics, New York, 1972, Appleton-Century-Crofts.
8. Easson, W. M.: The dying child, Springfield, Ill., 1970, Charles C Thomas, Publisher.
9. Evans, A. E., and Edin, S.: If a child must die, New England Journal of Medicine **278:**138-142, Jan. 18, 1968.
10. Fond, K. I.: Dealing with death and dying through family center care, Nursing

Clinics of North America **7:**53-64, March, 1972.
11. Friedman, S. B., and others: Childhood leukemia: a pamphlet for parents, Washington, D.C., 1972, U.S. Government Printing Office.
12. Green, M.: Care of the dying child, Pediatrics **40**(supp.):492-497, Sept., 1967.
13. Hamovitch, M. B.: The parent and the fatally ill child, Los Angeles, 1964, Delmar Publishing Co., Inc.
14. Holland, J. F., and Frei, E., III, editors: Cancer medicine, Philadelphia, 1974, Lea & Febiger.
15. Holland, J. F., and Glidewell, O.: Oncologists' reply: survival expectancy in acute lymphocytic leukemia, New England Journal of Medicine **287:**769-777, Oct. 12, 1972.
16. Kaplan, D.: Leukemia strains emotional ties, Medical World News, April 6, 1973.
17. Lampkin, B. C., McWilliams, N. B., and Mauer, A. M.: Treatment of acute leukemia, Pediatric Clinics of North America **19:**1123-1140, Nov., 1972.
18. Levine, A. S., Graw, R. G., and Young, R. C.: Management of infections in patients with leukemia and lymphoma: current concepts and experimental approaches, Seminars in Hematology **9:**141-179, April, 1972.
19. Mengel, C. E., Frei, E., III, and Nachman, R.: Hematology: principles and

---

*Available only to participating institutions from Children's Cancer Study Group Statistical Center, Los Angeles, Calif.

practice, Chicago, 1972, Year Book Medical Publishers, Inc.

20. Nathan, D. G., and Oski, F. A.: Hematology of infancy and childhood, Philadelphia, 1974, W. B. Saunders Co.

21. Petrillo, M., and Sanger, S.: Emotional care of hospitalized children, Philadelphia, 1972, J. B. Lippincott Co.

22. Pochedly, C.: Management of central nervous system leukemia in childhood, Clinical Pediatrics **11:**503-508, Sept., 1972.

23. Simone, J.: Acute lymphocytic leukemia in childhood, Seminars in Hematology **11:**25-39, Jan., 1974.

24. Simone, J. V., Holland, E., and Johnson, W.: Fatalities during remission of childhood leukemia, Blood **39:**759-770, June, 1972.

25. Sutow, W. W., Vietti, T., and Fernbach, D. J.: Clinical pediatric oncology, St. Louis, 1973, The C. V. Mosby Co.

26. Weetman, R. M., and Baehner, R. L.: Management of acute leukemia, Current Problems in Pediatrics **3:**1-52, Aug., 1973.

ASSESSMENT FORM: INTRACRANIAL TUMORS

Name   **Diagnosis**
Age   **Understanding, feelings about illness**

Vital signs: B/P_____ Pulse_____ Respirations_____ Temperature_____

Neurological status

Level of consciousness

Response to name: alert and appropriate
Ability to cooperate and follow directions
Orientation to environment
Response to touch, pain
Purposeful protective bodily responses
Deep tendon reflexes
Decerebrate, decorticate positioning

Cranial nerves

Eyes: PERRLA, EOM, corneal reflex
Cough, gag reflex both sides of posterior pharynx
Shows teeth, protrudes tongue
Frowns, smiles

Increased intracranial pressure

Impaired mentation, memory
Change in personality
Lethargy
Paresis, paralysis, ulnar drift
Dysphasia, aphasia
Changes in visual field or acuity
Changes in oculomotor control
Dizziness
Headache, seizures
Vomiting, nausea
Papilledema

10 Perspective on patient prognosis for realistic goal setting with primary and metastatic intracranial malignancies

MARGIE J. Van METER
CONSTANCE MARY CLARK

The methods of treating patients with brain tumor (either malignant or metastatic) have not changed significantly over the last few years, and therefore the prognosis of these patients is still poor. Life expectancy is in months rather than years, and the patient's functional ability usually deteriorates rapidly.[6]

This chapter will focus on the nature and treatment response of tumors and on the nursing care of the patient. Nursing articles will be cited as references for the oncology nurse without experience in neurologic monitoring and care of the patient with neurologic deficits.

Regardless of the patient's phase of illness (diagnostic, operative, recurrent) or tumor type (benign, malignant, metastatic), the nursing care is essentially the same. Only malignant tumors are included in this discussion, but what is true of them is also true of the benign tumor if it is not surgically accessible or if a benign glial cell becomes malignant. The intensity will vary but increased intracranial pressure, neurologic deficits, and fear of dying remain the basic problems.

Few oncologic nursing publications include a chapter on brain tumors, and the phrase "cancer of the brain" is not commonly used. The reasons may be the variable natural history of brain tumors and the low percentage of cancer deaths caused by brain tumors. Brain tumors account for approximately 2% of the deaths from all cancers.[15]

BIOLOGIC NATURE OF BRAIN TUMORS

The patient's prognosis is a legitimate and necessary concern of the nurse. It is an essential factor in all situations for realistic goal setting and planning. The histologic diagnosis is only one factor in predicting the patient's prognosis. The concept of benign versus malignant, when referring to brain tumors, is different from benign and malignant tumors elsewhere in the body. A brain tumor is considered benign if it is surgically accessible and if there are well-differentiated cells. Conversely, a brain tumor is considered malignant if it is surgically inaccessible or if the cells are not differentiated. The lack of space for a tumor to expand within the rigid skull causes pressure disturbances capable of resulting in death.

Table 4. Malignancy of intracranial tumors

Benign	Moderate		Malignant
	Differentiated	*Dedifferentiated*	
Meningioma	Astrocytoma I $\longrightarrow$	II III	Glioblastoma
Neurinoma	Ependymoma I $\longrightarrow$	II III	multiforme III, IV
Pituitary adenoma	Oligodendroglioma $\longrightarrow$	Oligodendro-	Medulloblastoma
Craniopharyngioma		blastoma	Metastatic
Colloid cyst			

Since surgically inaccessible benign tumors cause pressure disturbances, a benign tumor may be considered malignant because of location. Malignant means "causing or likely to cause death."

The biologic activity of the tumor is dependent on the basic cell type from which it originates. For example, tumors of the glial cells may eventually become dedifferentiated and highly malignant (glioblastoma multiforme) if they are not malignant initially. The tumors classified as moderately malignant (Table 4) have such a potential.

Since glial cells form the deeper brain structure, there are more gliomas in the deep areas of the brain, and the corpus callosum is frequently involved[8]. The corpus callosum is a huge commissure connecting many of the cortical areas of the two hemispheres.

Tumor growth is by expansion, infiltration, or a combination of the two. Benign tumors usually grow by expansion, that is, by enlargement around a central core, and tend to be encapsulated. Gliomas characteristically grow by infiltration and spread into interstices of the tissues. Metastatic tumors tend to grow by expansion but may be infiltrative. The mechanism of growth is a major factor in determining the surgical resectability and therefore the degree of malignancy.

Growth of primary intracranial tumors is essentially a localized and regional neoplastic process, and extension is usually to the spinal canal and cord. Metastasis of primary brain tumors to areas outside the central nervous system is being reported. The reasons for this phenomenon may be the increased months of life and the greater number of patients having surgery and other therapy. The mechanism(s) of metastasis is not firmly established. Metastasis of brain tumors can be related to surgical intervention, especially multiple operations, and possibly to radiation.[19]

The clinician's ability to predict the biologic activity of a tumor remains limited at the present time. The astute nurse should remember that the individual patient may fall anywhere along the whole range of outcomes and can even defy statistical conclusions.

A variety of systems for classifying of brain tumors has appeared in the literature. The greater the number of histologic subdivisions, the more difficult it is to remember them for use as a factor in prognostication. For this reason Table 4 includes only the common tumors in three general classifications. The nurse who wishes more information about a particular tumor will find Mullen's book *Essentials of Neurosurgery for Students and Practitioners*[11] helpful.

Metastatic tumors to the brain come mainly from bronchogenic and breast carcinoma, in addition to cancer malignancies from a variety of other sites, such as kidney, stomach, intestine, and skin. The patient with bronchogenic carcinoma may seek medical help because of symptoms from the metastatic tumor to the brain and still have no symptoms related to the primary tumor in the lung. Neurologic symptoms from metastatic breast tumors usually occur some time after mastectomy. Metastatic tumors tend to occur in areas supplied by the terminal branches of the middle cerebral artery, which are located around the junction of the temporal, parietal, and occipital lobes. The tumor is usually located in surgically accessible areas, and there may be single or multiple lesions.

The clinical mainfestations of intracranial neoplasms are dependent on the location and size of the tumor and on the presence and rapidity of occurrence of increased intracranial pressure. The mechanisms of the manifestations are (1) destruction of brain tissue, (2) compression of neural structures, (3) alterations in blood supply to neurons, (4) alterations in neuronal excitability, (5) increase in mass within the rigid skull, and (6) obstruction in cerebrospinal fluid circulation.[11]

The resulting symptom(s) may be impaired mentation or memory, change in personality, lethargy, paresis/paralysis, dysphasia/aphasia, changes in visual fields, acuity, or oculomotor muscles, seizure, headache, nausea and vomiting, and papilledema.

DIAGNOSTIC METHODS

The diagnostic methods available for investigation of suspected intracranial lesions have become more precise, but the patient's history and neurologic examination are still essential for early detection and for appropriate selection of diagnostic procedures. Skull x-ray films and laminograms, electroencephalograms, brain scans, EMI scans, lumbar punctures, cerebral arteriograms, and pneumoencephalograms are now available. The usual sequence of diagnostic procedures in nonemergency situations is from the innocuous to those with a potential for associated morbidity. The progression is also to a more specific delineation of location, size, and structures involved.

A British-built machine called an EMI scanner may eventually replace the nuclear brain scan. The EMI machine scans sections of the brain 1 cm wide and, with computer assistance, produces pictures with detail sufficient to distinguish between stroke and tumor and to measure depth of the tumor. It is not uncomfortable, neither is it hazardous. The patient lies prone, with the head in a small rubber cap, while an x-ray tube moves over the head in semicircles. The full diagnostic potential with the EMI scanner has not yet been fully determined. The other diagnostic procedures are discussed in basic nursing texts. At University Hospital, guidelines for physical preparation and for aftercare of the patient have been printed on 2½ × 3 inch slips and are clipped to the Kardex the day the

---

NAME
Pneumoencephalogram
               on _____ at _____

Prep: Aftercare:
1. Permit obtained by physician.   1. SCB for 24 hours.
2. NPO after midnight.   2. Ice cap prn for headache.
3. On call medication as ordered.   3. Bed flat for 24 hours.
4. Patient to wear hospital gown. Re-   4. Vital signs and pupil check as or-
   move dentures, hairpins, etc.   dered.
5. Transport on stretcher.   5. Resume medications and treatments
6. Take medical record and addresso-   unless ordered otherwise.
   graph card.   6. Diet as tolerated.
        (Front)   *(Back)*

---

study is to be done. (See example above.*) Similar forms are available for all diagnostic procedures.

The informational needs related to diagnostic studies are primarily related to the sensations the patient will experience: "How will it feel?" Cautioning the patient that a warm sensation, which is caused by the injected arteriogram dye and the tilting and maneuvering of the pneumochair, can be expected helps the patient remain calm. More complete information for patient preparation can be found in articles by Blackwell[2] and by Sheaver and Creel.[14]

Asking the patient and/or family whether they have heard of anyone who has had the test elicits their degree of understanding and makes it possible to clarify any misconceptions. For example, a woman scheduled for arteriography said that she was very fearful because another patient had told her about being unconscious for 3 days after an arteriogram. In fact, the other patient had not been unconscious but because of her psychiatric problem described herself as such. To promote consistency in informing patients about diagnostic studies and to evaluate the patient's understanding, a patient education checklist is used for neurosurgery patients at University Hospital. (See example on pp. 123 and 124.)

NEUROLOGIC MONITORING

The intracranial pressure may be at a borderline level from the tumor mass and increasing cerebral edema. Since acute embarrassment of cranial structures and functions can occur, close neurologic monitoring is needed. A critical indicator of neurologic function is the level of consciousness. It is more precise to describe the patient's responses than to use labels, since a patient is rarely at a discrete level of consciousness, and examiners vary in their interpretation of the labels. There are two components to consider and record regarding patient responses: (1) the amount and type of stimulus needed to elicit a response, and (2) the type and

---

*Courtesy University of Michigan Medical Center, Department of Nursing, Ann Arbor, Mich.

NURSING—PATIENT EDUCATION CHECKLIST*

Prediagnostic procedures	Test to be done ($\surd$)	Patient taught Date	Patient taught By	Asked questions on back of sheet patient correctly answered (initial) A	B	C	D	Date test completed
Blood survey admission	___	___	___	___	___	___	___	___
Urinalysis admission	___	___	___	___	___	___	___	___
Chest x-ray	___	___	___	___	___	___	___	___
Skull x-ray	___	___	___	___	___	___	___	___
Brain scan	___	___	___	___	___	___	___	___
EEG	___	___	___	___	___	___	___	___
ECG	___	___	___	___	___	___	___	___
Arteriogram	___	___	___	___	___	___	___	___
Pneumoen-cephalogram	___	___	___	___	___	___	___	___
EMI	___	___	___	___	___	___	___	___
Spinal x-ray	___	___	___	___	___	___	___	___
Laminagram	___	___	___	___	___	___	___	___
Myelogram	___	___	___	___	___	___	___	___
Audiogram	___	___	___	___	___	___	___	___
	___	___	___	___	___	___	___	___
	___	___	___	___	___	___	___	___

Preoperative: Patient aware surgery for _____ is planned on _____

(signed) _____

	Patient taught Date	By	Patient demonstrated Date	To	Patient stated Date	One purpose To
Deep breathing/coughing	___	___	___	___	___	___
Leg exercises	___	___	___	___	___	___
Jobst stockings	___	___			___	___
Tubes	___	___			___	___
Nothing by mouth	___	___			___	___
Premedication	___	___			___	___
Recovery room/special care area	___	___			___	___
Family waiting room	___	___			___	___
Postoperative monitoring routines	___	___			___	___
Postoperative activity allowed	___	___			___	___
Postoperative comfort measures	___	___			___	___

Predischarge: Patient expects to go _____ on _____

(signed) _____

Statement of patient (day of discharge) in reference to:
Activity restrictions: _____
Care of incision: _____
Medications: _____
Medical/nursing follow-up: _____

(signed) _____

(Front)

*Courtesy University of Michigan Medical Center, Department of Nursing, October, 1974.

extent of the response. The losing and regaining of alert oriented consciousness occur on a continuum. The intensity of stimulation required to elicit a response as the level of consciousness deteriorates occurs on a continuum from the absence of stimuli with spontaneous behavior to stimuli required to elicit any response, and from verbal stimuli to tactile stimuli to painful stimuli. The descending order of responses is: alert and appropriate responses; ability to inability to cooperate and follow directions; orientation to disorientation; purposeful protective bodily responses to purposeless movements; presence to absence of cough and corneal reflexes; and no response. Gardner[5] and Salibi[13] give more detail in their articles.

Detecting subtle changes in responsiveness may require comparison over a period of time. The problem-oriented patient record makes this information more quickly retrievable, and for this reason the neurosurgical nursing staff of University Hospital adapted problem-oriented charting to better monitor their patients. The neurologic monitoring of a patient with a tumor includes assessment of the level of consciousness, vital signs, motor strength, and pupillary reflexes. Observation of ulnar drift is a means of detecting the presence of slight hemiparesis. The patient is instructed to close eyes and outstretch both arms in front, with the palms up. Paresis will cause the elbow to flex and the hand to turn inward. A quick check of cranial nerves and the pupillary reflex can be made by having the patient look in all four quadrants, show the teeth, frown, smile, and protrude the tongue, and by stimulating both sides of the posterior pharynx for gag reflex. A detailed guide for nurses to the neurologic examination is given by Van Meter and Diehl.[18]

Level of consciousness, vital signs, motor function, and reflexes are indirect indicators of intracranial pressure. The intracranial pressure screw is a means of direct measurement. A screw is placed through the skull and duramater into the cerebrospinal fluid in the subarachnoid space. The intracranial pressure can then be measured by following the principles used for measuring central venous pressure. Tilbury[17] gives more information about the intracranial pressure screw.

MANAGEMENT OF CEREBRAL EDEMA

Edematous brain tissue surrounds many brain tumors, especially the fast-growing gliomas and metastatic tumors. Marked edema extends for a considerable distance and occasionally into the opposite hemisphere. Cerebral edema is reflected in papilledema. Therapy to relieve the symptoms of the preoperative patient or the one with a nonoperative malignancy is based on relieving the pressure caused by edema. Dexamethasone, hyperosmolar therapy, fluid restriction, and head elevation help to attain this goal. Dexamethasone, a potent synthetic adrenocortical steroid, relieves symptoms by its effect on the edematous brain and thus decreases brain bulk and intracranial pressure. An initial dose of 10 mg. is followed by a 5- to 7-day taper beginning with 4 mg./6 hr and decreasing to the smallest dose necessary to control symptoms. Tapering is necessary to avoid exacerbation of edema with sudden withdrawal and relative adrenal insufficiency after a week of dexamethasone therapy. It is relatively free of other side effects except on the gastrointestinal tract. Antacids are given as concomitant preventive therapy. The remission of symptoms does much for the patient's confidence in the physician preoperatively because improvement is evident.

Mannitol is replacing urea as the hyperosmolar substance used for cerebral dehydration in acute situations. Hyperosmolar agents draw fluid from the brain to the vascular space and cause diuresis.

Fluid intake is restricted to a minimal daily requirement range, usually 1000 to 1500 ml./24 hr. Confused patients require creative measures, such as covering the faucets to prevent the drinking of undesirable amounts of fluids. However, nausea and vomiting caused by the malignant process may result in dehydration. Close monitoring of the patient is needed while hydration, especially by the intravenous route, is established. As the body is hydrated, so is the edematous brain tissue, and acute decompensation can result. In one instance a patient died on

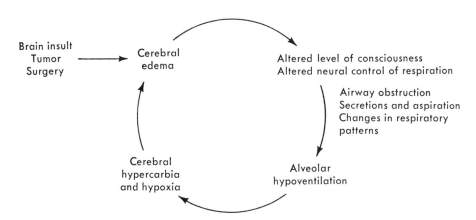

Fig. 3. Cycle of deterioration created by brain insult and inadequate respiratory function.

the night before surgery from the attempt to establish hydration for the operation. The brain absorbed too much of the fluid, and acute intracranial pressure resulted.

Elevating the head of the bed is an attempt to affect the edema by using gravity to promote venous return from the brain. Venous circulation from the cranium is retarded by raised intrathoracic venous pressure.

Cerebral hypercapnia and hypoxia have an adverse effect on brain edema and intracranial pressure. Ventilatory assistance or control is a potent and readily used means of reducing intracranial pressure when acute brain lesions with associated edema exist. Brain insult and inadequate respiratory function create a cycle of deterioration.[12] This cycle is simplified and diagrammed in Fig. 3.

Pulmonary toilet, a patent airway, and assisted ventilation are sometimes prophylactic, and urgent in other situations. Measures must be instituted immediately once they are determined to be necessary. Periodic arterial blood gas determinations evaluate effectiveness of the therapy.

BRAIN TUMOR THERAPIES

Surgical intervention of accessible tumors is done to decompress the tumor bulk and remove necrotic brain tissue. A rapidly growing tumor causes central necrosis by cutting off its own blood supply. Necrotic brain tissue has a deleterious effect on the function of the surrounding hemisphere or brain stem. Truely radical excision is rarely attempted because functioning areas would be compromised. If the tumor's location and malignant nature prevent removal, the objectives are to remove as much tumor as possible, preserve as much function as possible, relieve symptoms, and prolong life.

Recurrent cerebral tumors require decisions similar to those made at the time of the initial occurrence. Should the treatment consist of surgical exploration with the intention of resecting more tumor; steroid therapy to relieve symptoms; insertion of a shunt for blocked flow of cerebrospinal fluid; or the use of analgesics, sedatives, and tranquilizers for pain and anxiety until consciousness is depressed by the tumor?

The impact of radiotherapeutic methods on longevity with a brain tumor has been limited to a few tumor types such as pituitary adenoma and medulloblastoma. The aim of ionizing radiation treatment is to destroy tumor cells without killing normal neural tissue. It is now increasingly believed that radiation that is destructive to tumor cells must be given in doses close to tolerance of the normal brain cells, since the brain is not as radioresistant as once believed.[19] Sophisticated apparatus with beam directional equipment that allows for precision is essential to limit the effect to the tumor area. A delayed effect of radiation on the brain is necrosis, usually of white matter and the brain stem. Whole brain radiation may be used for tumors when long-term survival is not expected.

The pathology report, natural history of the tumor if untreated, tumor location, extent of neurologic deficit, and general health are factors in deciding to what extent normal brain tissue should be placed in jeopardy by radiation for the sake of tumor suppression or destruction. The variable natural history of brain tumors adds complexity to the decision and confusion about statistical results of specific modes of therapy.

Because of the variable natural history of brain tumors and the variable response to radiation of specific cell types, it is impossible to make an accurate prognosis. However, since the nurse who is helping the patient and family establish realistic goals needs some clues as to the possible effect radiation may have on prognosis, the more common results for tumor types are listed below.[6,10]

Astrocytoma I and II	Relatively good prognosis from surgery without irradiation
Ependymoma	Postoperative radiation, 58% to 87% 5-year survival
Oligodendroglioma	Postoperative radiation, 85% 5-year survival
Medulloblastoma	Postoperative radiation, 25% to 30% 5-year survival
Glioblastoma multiforme	Palliative-50% symptom relief radiation with BCNU chemotherapy
Metastatic	Palliative-63% symptom relief with whole brain radiation if cannot localize

Radiation is given after craniotomy so that treatment can be rationally based on histologic proof. For the nurse, there are two areas of concern associated with radiotherapy. It should be stressed to the patient and family that consultation with the radiotherapist is done to decide whether radiotherapy is an appropriate treatment. Focusing on the value of radiation therapy before the radiotherapist's decision is known raises hopes and may cause unnecessary anxiety.

Transient reactions occasionally occur with radiotherapy. The reaction thought to be from radiation-produced brain edema causes symptoms similar to those of the original tumor. The patient usually begins therapy before discharge so that he can be observed during initial treatment.

Chemotherapy for brain malignancies has lagged behind chemotherapy for other types of malignancies. Neurotoxicity of structures vital to life and the blood-brain barrier phenomenon are part of the reason. The blood-brain barrier is a physiologic, not an anatomic, barrier around each cell of brain substance that protects the cell from noxious substances. There is a selective permeability to substances between the capillary and the brain cell, but a brain insult can change the barrier's permeability. To be clinically effective, a cancer drug must have properties that permit it to cross the normal blood-brain barrier or alter the normal permeability of the blood-tumor barrier.

Trial and error based on remission and nonrecurrence of symptoms have been the guides for chemotherapy. The rapid growth of glioblastoma and its associated edema, which may be the cause of symptom recurrence, does not permit accurate results from the trial-and-error method. Tumor size as a measurement of drug effectiveness has not been possible as with cancer in other areas. Cerebral arteriography and the brain scan do not distinguish between tumor and edematous brain, and therefore the size of the tumor cannot be measured. Studies that measure effectiveness by treated and untreated survival are needed. For patients with glioblastoma survival must be for at least 18 months.

Glioblastoma multiforme is the major central nervous system malignancy in which new chemotherapeutic agents are currently being tested. The results of a randomized prospective study of the Brain Tumor Study Group under the sponsorship of the National Cancer Institute suggests that the drug BCNU and irradiation will lengthen patient survival with malignant glioma.[4] Palliation was shown in approximately 50% of treated patients. BCNU, MeCCNU, and CCNU are nitrosourea drugs. They are highly lipid-soluble and thus may be capable of permeating the blood-brain barrier. All are being studied, along with a variety modes of administration such as carotid artery infusion and ventricular instillation. Methotrexate administered intrathecally and vincristine administered intravenously have an effect on medulloblastoma, but they, too, fail to achieve cures.

ASPECTS OF NURSING CARE

Certain commonalities of nursing care are necessary for the patient with a malignant or metastatic brain tumor regardless of the phase of the illness: diagnostic, operative, or recurrent. Since the majority of patients do undergo surgery, consisting of either gross total removal or debulking and biopsy to identify cell type, this discussion will focus primarily on the operative phase. However, the same principles, depending on the patient's functional abilities, apply to the patient who is not a candidate for surgery. A discussion of such functional deficits as weakness, spatial dysfunction, aphasia, and balance problems is found in the article "Adapting Care for the Brain-Damaged Patient."[4]

The concept of malfunction of brain cells is frightening to many and is associated with fear of dependency, serious functional disabilities, alteration of daily living patterns, and ultimate doom. The diagnosis of malignant or metastatic brain tumor is particularly devastating to the patient and the family. They frequently exhibit the behavior described by Kübler-Ross in *On Death and Dying*[9]*:* anger, bargaining, depression, and acceptance.

The focus of the patient with a brain tumor seems to be the fear of loss of control and the fear of being a burden to the family. Anger may be expressed, particularly if the patient is in the productive time of life. If the tumor has metastasized from an already diagnosed primary site, feelings of "having suffered enough" may be verbalized. If the patient's symptoms include deterioration of mental faculties or personality change, family and friends may be irritated and embarrassed by the behavior. Subsequently, they may feel guilt for their expression of anger. The patient and family may also openly express the hope for a miracle or the hope that the pathologic diagnosis was incorrect. The nurse should attempt to support the family at their level of functioning. The family can be assisted by listening and by helping them set short-term, achievable goals.

If surgery is the treatment of choice, preoperative teaching may be difficult. The patient may not be aware enough to understand explanations, and the family's anxiety may be too great to comprehend details. However, the patient and the family need explanations, however simplified. The content of the teaching depends on their comprehension.

The patient may not be capable, at first, of reacting directly to the diagnosis of brain tumor and may express anxiety in other ways. A commonly observed reaction is excessive concern and frequent prolonged lamentation about the need for the head to be shaved prior to surgery. It can be therapeutic for the patient to initially express his fears by talking about the head shaving. However, after surgery, it is rare for a patient to express much concern or demonstrate particular modesty about the ½-inch long hair once the head dressing is removed. It is as if the heavy weight of fear associated with the craniotomy is lessened, and the immediate actual concerns become important. Postoperative craniotomy patients benefit from the current "bald is beautiful" image of Telly Savalas, society's generally freer hair styling, and the wig fad. Once women had wigs brought to the hospital before surgery for wearing at the first opportunity after surgery. One woman had twelve wigs lined up in her room on the day of surgery. Today frilly boudoir caps are worn, with little concern expressed about obtaining a wig.

Safety is an important aspect of care. Nursing concern with safety includes medicolegal considerations in addition to patient well-being. The current drastic increase in the number of lawsuits against physicians, hospitals, and nurses has made physicians and nurses extremely wary and perhaps overzealous in their concern about safety. Patients with brain tumors may have deficiencies in balance or judgment. Consequently, they are more prone to falls. The nurse must constantly provide for the safety of the patient without being excessive in attempts to prevent falls. Attendance for bathroom and ambulation activities and vest restraints are therapeutic only if the nurse provides for activity and change of position.

Usually the family members cooperate with nursing actions to provide safety when they are helped to understand that the measures are precautionary to prevent injury, and are not punishments. The family's presence and watchful eyes may be used as an opportunity to remove restraints for more freedom of movement.

Placing a piece of extra tubing in the hands of a confused patient sometimes serves as a distraction, so that he will not pull on other tubing, such as urinary drainage tubing. Interval voiding encourages continence and discourages climbing of side rails. Physical activity, that is, chair sitting and ambulation, reduce the tendency of the patient to get out of bed without supervision.

The unconscious patient can be gotten out of bed to reduce the sequela of immobility. A sturdy chair with a high back and arm support is needed. If there is poor head control, the head can be kept upright by tying a stretch gauze around the forehead (avoiding the eyes) and the back of the chair.

Some patients may have difficulty urinating because of their short attention span and need constant reminders. Patients may have less difficulty with incontinence or retention if they are taken to the bathroom instead of using a bedpan or urinal. Interval voiding is no joy for either patient or nurse, but it is a workable method for patients to relearn how to use the toilet. Some patients may need additional stimulus to void, such as the icing and brushing techniques described in "Sensory Stimulation Techniques."[16]

The nurse should attempt to reorient the patient through use of the familiar. The unfamiliar hospital environment, the extraneous noises, the changes in diurnal routine, and the strangers in white uniforms tend to increase the confusion of the patient. Pictures of family and friends, personal clothing instead of the standard shapeless hospital gown, tub baths, and favorite foods all contribute meaningful stimuli to the disoriented patient.

Because of the nature and symptoms of the illness, the patient may suffer sensory deprivation. Too often, the patient has little contact with anyone except staff and family. Discriminating use of the radio or television can help to stimulate sensory input. The nurse should seek information about the patient's likes and dislikes, and should encourage the watching or listening of programs that are meaningful and entertaining to the patient. A radio or television that is constantly turned on is not positive sensory input.

After a craniotomy, the scalp is particularly itchy as the hair starts to grow in. The nurse may be confronted with a patient who repeatedly pulls off the head dressing to scratch. Scratching of the incision predisposes the patient to the dangers of a wound infection, which can result in osteomyelitis or brain abscess. Consequently, craniotomy incisions are covered until sutures are out and the wound is healed. Well-secured head dressing that is replaced promptly if it is pulled off, as well as trimmed fingernails and bulky mittens or arm restraints, may be necessary if the patient is unable to remember not to scratch. Washing the hair at the earliest approved time helps to reduce the itching sensation.

Corneal ulceration is a potential problem if the patient is unable to completely close one or both eyes due to decreased level of consciousness or facial nerve paralysis. Special care is needed if the eyelid does not cover the iris completely when the eye is closed. Likewise, sluggish or absent corneal reflexes require special care. The patient may not be aware that a foreign object is in the eye or that the cornea is drying, and infection or ulceration may result. Preventive care includes the instillation of artificial tears, the closing of the eye, and eye patching. Instillation of the eye drops lubricates the eye. Two methods are used to close the eye. First, the eye may be taped shut and/or an eye patch applied over the eye. Eye patch application must assure the continued closure of the eye, since the gauze could irritate the cornea. The tape is removed at least daily by starting from top to bottom of the tape and by avoiding undue pull on the eyelashes. Exudates around the eye are removed, the eye is examined for moistness and signs of redness, and new tape and/or an eye patch is reapplied.

The second method used to close the eye is tarsorrhaphy, the suturing together of part or all of the upper and lower eyelids. Again, eye care is needed to prevent encrustation around the eyelid. Tarsorrhaphy is frequently done in the absence of corneal reflex or cranial nerve palsy if the condition is expected to continue for a prolonged time.

The nurse may be concerned with fever control, particularly after surgery. Frequently, aspirin or acetaminophen (Tylenol) and hypothermia are sufficient to lower the temperature, but sponging may be necessary for a severe fever spike of 105° to 106° F. Fever increases the metabolic and oxygen needs of the brain. The objective is to lower body temperature without causing the patient to shiver, since shivering increases body temperature and intracranial pressure. Sponging is most effective if a mixture of warm water and alcohol is used in conjunction with massage. The warm water and massage produce vasodilation, and the alcohol cools by evaporation. The nurse should remove a hypothermia blanket before sponging to prevent frostbite to the patient from the moisture and cold blanket. The patient's body temperature is related to the temperature of the room and the number of blankets covering him. Judicious use of bed linens can prevent fever spikes. The family needs an explanation of why the patient has no blankets.

Headache continues to be an aggravating problem throughout the course of the illness. The headache usually responds to relatively mild analgesics such as aspirin or codeine. Normally, comfort measures such as heating pad, cool cloths, or massage have little added effect, since the physiologic cause of the headache, the increased pressure on the internal structures of the brain and blood vessels in the brain, is not influenced by them. Elevation of the head of the bed may reduce the headache because the effect of gravity decreases the pressure within the skull.

The nursing care of the patient with a malignant or metastatic tumor includes provision for the present and planning for the future. Typically, the patient will be discharged from the hospital after optimum treatment has been initiated or accomplished. The patient and/or family must decide where and by whom the disabled patient will be cared for after discharge. A coordinated approach with nurse, physician, and social worker helps the family to learn the alternatives and helps to support them in their decisions. The physician informs about prognosis, and the nurse reviews the care the patient requires, exploring with the family their ability to provide the care at home and teaching the care to the families that make the decision for home care. The social worker also assists the family with their decision making and with locating an extended care facility if that is their decision. The family needs clear information about any insurance for home and extended care coverage. If skilled supervision and care by a visiting nurse is not indicated at the time of discharge, the family should nevertheless be aware that community agencies are available for assistance and support. The nurse and social worker can provide information about available resources. The hospital nurse should communicate sufficient information on the assessment, goals, and care of the patient to enable the visiting nurse to provide continuity of care. The visiting nurse should be aware of the rationale for treatment and of the expected course of the disease. To communicate efficiently with the visiting nurse and at the same time complete the inpatient nursing record, make a carbon copy of the referral and place it on the inpatient record. Predischarge teaching is necessary even if discharge must be postponed until the teaching has been completed. The family should feel confident to care for the patient at the time of discharge. If the patient has hemiparesis, the family should have basic information about assisting him to move, dress, and eat. If the patient is to be discharged with catheter or condom drainage, the family should understand the rationale for, and care of, the equipment. If the patient has poor balance or muscular coordination, the nurse may suggest rearrangement of furniture in the house. She may also suggest that the family acquire such equipment as a walker, bedpan, or vest restraint.

The most successful discharge planning incorporates the extended family and community to assist with the care of the patient. Frequently, the care needs of the patient are too taxing for one person to handle, but they are manageable with assistance. For example, grown sons or neighbors can help the patient get out of bed, and neighbors can assist with grocery shopping.

This extensive preparation may be done, and then the patient is at home for only a brief period of 10 to 14 days. The time invested for family preparation was appropriate. When the patient and/or family desire home care, no matter how brief, the opportunity should be available. It can do much for family comfort by avoiding guilt reactions.

The family of the patient who is to enter an extended care facility may feel guilty that they are unable to care for the patient. The nurse should reinforce positive aspects of placement, stressing that the nursing home is equipped to meet the needs of the convalescent patient. If the facility is located closer to the family than the hospital, this advantage should be mentioned.

As the disease progresses, the patient may be readmitted to the hospital for terminal care. The physician will discuss with the family the decision to avoid further aggressive treatment. The goal of nursing, therefore, is to provide comfort for the patient and support to the family. As the patient becomes more obtunded, the family should be reassured that there is no pain. The patient's respiratory pattern frequently becomes noisy and grotesque; positioning the patient on the side or inserting an oral airway often minimizes the sound. If the family feels that getting the patient out of bed is difficult and nontherapeutic, the nurse should re-evaluate the plan of care. Nursing actions may need to be changed to ensure that the goal of provision of comfort is achieved.

As the patient becomes terminal, the family must be kept informed. They should be permitted to see the bedside vital signs graphic if that is helpful for them. The vital signs and overall status should be interpreted so that the family can make decisions to stay at the bedside or to leave. If the family telephones for information on the patient's condition, the nurse should courteously give them information about the patient that they would observe if they were at the bedside, for example, level of response, any food or fluid intake, state of comfort, or elevated temperature.

The nurse can be valuable support to the family as the patient's condition deteriorates. With knowledge of the disease process, methods of diagnosis and treatment, and outcome, the nurse can plan comprehensive patient care. Often, the nurse has cared for the patient during a previous admission, knows and relates to the family, and can extend comfort and dignity to the circumstances.

REFERENCES

1. Belt, L.: Working with dysphasic patients, American Journal of Nursing **74:** 1320-1322, July, 1974.
2. Blackwell, C. A.: PEG and angiography: a patient's sensations, American Journal of Nursing **75:**264-266, Feb., 1975.
3. Erickson, R.: Cranial check: a basic neurological assessment, Nursing '74, pp. 67-72, Aug., 1974.
4. Fowler, R. S., and Fordyce, W. E.: Adapting care for the brain-damaged patient, American Journal of Nursing **72:** 1832-1835, 2056-2059, Nov., 1972.
5. Gardner, A. M.: Responsiveness as a measure of consciousness, American Journal of Nursing **68:** 1035-1038, May, 1968.
6. Goldsmith, M. A., and Carter, S. K.: Glioblastoma multiforme: a review of therapy, Cancer Treatment Review **1:** 153-165,
7. Gray, R.: Grief, Nursing '74, pp. 25-27, Jan., 1974.
8. Kahn, E. A., and others: Correlative neurosurgery, Springfield, Ill., 1969, Charles C Thomas, Publisher.
9. Kübler-Ross, E.: On death and dying, New York, 1969, The Macmillan Co.
10. Moss, W. T., Brand, W. N., and Battifora, H.: Radiation oncology: rationale, technique, results, ed. 4, St. Louis, 1973, The C. V. Mosby Co.
11. Mullen, S.: Essential of neurosurgery for students and practitioners, New York, 1961, Springer Publishing Co., Inc.
12. Parsons, L. C.: Respiratory changes in head injury, American Journal of Nursing **71:**2187-2191, Dec., 1971.
13. Salibi, B. S.: Levels of consciousness, The Wisconsin Medical Journal, pp. 375-377, Sept., 1963.
14. Sheaver, D., and Creel, D.: Preparing the patient for EEG, American Journal of Nursing **75:**63-64, Jan., 1975.
15. Silverberg, E., and Holleb, A. I.: Cancer statistics 1973, Cancer **23:**1-27, 1973.
16. Sister Regina Elizabeth: Sensory stimulation techniques, American Journal of Nursing **66:**281-286, Feb., 1966.
17. Tilbury, M. S.: The intracranial pressure screw: a new assessment tool, Nursing Clinics of North America **9:**4, 641-646, Dec., 1974.
18. Van Meter, M. J., and Diehl, E.: Detection of alterations in neuromuscular functioning. In Sana, J. M., and Judge, R. D., editors: Physical appraisal methods in nursing practice, Boston, 1975, Little, Brown & Co.
19. Youmans, J. R., editor: Neurological surgery vol 3, Philadelphia, 1973, W. B. Saunders Co.

ASSESSMENT FORM: LUNG CANCER

Name   **Understanding**
Age   **Diagnosis**   **and feelings**
Sex   **Previous history of cancer**   **about illness**

Respiratory status

Occupation (presence of air pollutants)
History of smoking
Chest x-ray examination
Intermittent cough lasting longer than 2 to 3 weeks
S.O.B., wheezing, respiratory rate
History of respiratory problems: emphysema, bronchitis
Sputum production
Hemoptysis
Chest pain, poorly localized ache
Hoarseness
Edema of face, neck, and upper extremities
Dysphagia

Systemic symptoms

Weakness, weight loss, malaise
Secondary infection: chills, fever, night sweats
Clubbing of fingers and toes
Arthralgia 2° hypertrophy of distal ends of long bones
Vertigo, dementia, paresthesia
↑ADH
Metabolic disorders; signs of Cushing's syndrome
Changes in lymph nodes

11 Nursing the patient with lung cancer

SUSAN LYNN ZIMMERMAN

Much research is presently being done to discover ways to prevent and to cure cancer. As this research continues, however, cancer of the lung has increased to nearly epidemic proportions. In one day nearly 200 persons succumb to this disease. It is the leading cause of deaths from cancer among men, and its incidence is increasing among women as they become habitual smokers. Furthermore, only one person in ten suffering from lung cancer is cured.[6] Even among those patients who are thought to have resectable lesions and who return home apparently cured, approximately one half to two thirds will die of the disease within 6 to 18 months.[4]

The distressing aspect of this disease is that it has been proved nearly beyond doubt in the Surgeon General's reports that cigarette smoking is the prime cause of lung cancer. Men smoking more than one pack of cigarettes a day are twenty times more likely to die of lung cancer than the nonsmoker.[1] The way to decrease the incidence of the disease would appear to be straightforward—yet the number of deaths increases.

Because of this alarming increase in the incidence of lung cancer, challenges are presented to the nursing profession in all areas along the health care continuum— from prevention of the disease to providing support and comfort to the patient whose disease is found to be inoperable.

This chapter will include a discussion of the development, growth, and spread of lung cancer. It will also deal with prevention and methods of diagnosis, surgical intervention, and palliative therapy. Utilization of the nursing process in caring for these patients will also be discussed. For a discussion of the pathophysiology of lung cancer, see Watson.[13]

PREVENTION

Since early detection of lung cancer presently remains very difficult, the only hope of extinguishing the disease seems to lie in prevention by educating the public not to smoke cigarettes. Nurses, who are employed in a variety of settings, can reach many population groups and should assume significant responsibility in educating the public regarding ways of preventing lung cancer.

The greatest increase in smoking recently has been in girls between 12 and 18 years of age. In 1968, 8.4% of this group were smokers. By 1972 the percentage had risen to 13.3%. Today, it is more important than ever for school nurses to educate the school-age population regarding the hazards of smoking.[8]

Nurses employed in industries where workers are exposed to carcinogenic

135

irritants need to be certain that these employees are aware of the symptoms of lung cancer and that they undergo regular health examinations.

Nurses in any setting, whether it be the community or the hospital, need to recognize situations in which persons need information regarding prevention of lung cancer. The American Cancer Society can be helpful to the nurse who is planning such teaching.

SYMPTOMS

Early diagnosis of lung cancer is mandatory if any hope for a cure is to be offered to the patient. Unfortunately, lung cancer in its early stages results in only minimal physiologic changes. These changes may produce either no symptoms or symptoms that are intermittent and do not alert the patient to seek medical help.[13]

In addition, diagnosis may be quite difficult in patients already suffering from a pulmonary disease such as chronic bronchitis or emphysema. Patients who are symptomatic from these diseases may have far-advanced cancer before the diagnosis is made.[1]

The symptoms that are produced by cancer of the lung are quite varied. They are related to the location of the tumor and to the rate and pattern of spread of the particular cell type. The initial symptoms are of a respiratory nature in about 50% of the patients. The others present with extrapulmonary symptoms or are alerted to the lung lesion by an incidental chest x-ray film or sputum test.[1]

The most common symptom of lung cancer is a cough. It may be insidious in onset, beginning during an upper respiratory infection but lasting long after the signs of the illness are gone. Therefore all coughs or other signs of respiratory infection that last longer than 2 to 3 weeks should be investigated by a physician.[6,13]

The mucosal and submucosal location of lung lesions accounts for the high frequency of this symptom. The tumor causes the surrounding mucous glands to oversecrete and stimulate coughing. Also, the vagal nerve endings are quite sensitive to the irritation produced by the swelling of the bronchial mucous membrane.[1,13]

The cough is at first most noticeable during the night or in the morning, becoming intermittent during the day. The cough may increase with exertion. It is generally nonproductive in the beginning, but later mucoid secretions are produced. If infection occurs due to an obstructed bronchus, purulent sputum is produced.[13]

If the larger bronchi are involved, the patient's cough becomes brassy with wheezing. Involvement of the mediastinal structures leads to a choking sensation, often precipitated by the patient's lying down. If the lesion has invaded the pleura, the cough is usually accompanied by a pleurisy type of pain that will disappear as a pleural effusion develops.[13]

One out of 4 persons over 40 years old who exhibits the symptom of hemoptysis has cancer. Hemoptysis occurs after ulceration of the bronchial mucous membrane or as the tumor causes erosion of the pulmonary blood vessels.[13]

The receptors of pain in the chest are limited to the nerve endings of the parietal pleura, the mediastinum, the trachea, and the large blood vessels of the thorax. The smaller bronchi are not sensitive to the usual pain stimuli. Consequently, pain in a patient with lung cancer is usually an ominous sign indicative of spread beyond the primary site.[1]

Ulceration of a bronchus may cause a dull, poorly localized ache in the chest. Pleuritic pain can be due to direct spread of the tumor to the pleura or because of atelectasis and pneumonia behind an obstructed bronchus. When lung cancer metastasizes to the bony structures of the chest wall, the patient experiences dull, unremitting pain with tenderness over the area. In addition, lung tumors that are located near the diaphragm may cause irritation of the phrenic nerve leading to referred pain in the shoulders.[1]

Although shortness of breath eventually occurs in most patients, it is rarely a presenting symptom in patients with lung neoplasms. Impaired respiration may occur as the tumor grows and displaces lung tissue, when atelectasis or pneumonia develops, or because of a pleural effusion.[1]

Hoarseness in patients with lung cancer is due to involvement of the recurrent laryngeal nerve.[3] Edema of the face, neck, and upper extremities is a sign that characterizes the superior vena cava syndrome and occurs when this vein becomes obstructed by the tumor. It is most often seen in patients with oat cell carcinoma. Difficulty in swallowing is noticed because the tumor presses against the esophagus.[13]

The systemic symptoms of weakness, weight loss, and malaise are caused by the shunting of nutrients to the neoplasm to meet its high energy requirements.[1] Infection secondary to an obstructed airway may cause additional generalized symptoms of chills, fever, and night sweat.[13]

Other extrathoracic symptoms often seen with lung cancer include clubbing of the toes and fingers and hypertrophy of the distal ends of the long bones, which causes arthralgia. Neurologic symptoms—such as vertigo, dementia, and paresthesia—may occur even without metastasis. The cause is uncertain. Metabolic disorders may develop, and the patient may exhibit signs of Cushing's syndrome. Excessive quantities of the antidiuretic hormone may be produced.[13]

In some instances the signs and symptoms that first cause the patient with a primary lung tumor to seek medical help are those due to metastatic spread of the cancer. All types of bronchogenic cancer tend to metastasize early. About 80% of the lesions are spread by the bloodstream, and the remaining 20% metastasize by way of the lymph. Oat cell carcinomas in particular metastasize rapidly.[4]

DIAGNOSIS OF CARCINOMA OF THE LUNG

When a person comes to a physician with signs and symptoms suggestive of a lung lesion, a number of examinations will be carried out to determine whether a malignancy of the lung does exist, and if so, the location and extent of the disease. The results of the data will then help the physician decide on the best type of treatment for the individual patient.

The nurse needs to be familiar with the diagnostic tests to be helpful in preparing the patient for the procedures. Careful preparation usually means that more reliable information will be obtained.

A thorough radiologic examination will be carried out initially on patients admitted to the hospital for an evaluation for lung cancer. From the x-ray examination the physician will attempt to define the pathology by interpreting patterns of increased or decreased density.

Posteroanterior and lateral films are taken to furnish information concerning the size of the tumor and its location. With these two films, a three-dimensional localization can be defined. Oblique views that are inclined at certain angles are taken to visualize the mediastinal structures, and lordotic films are taken to study the apices of the lungs. Decubitus films are taken with the patient in the lateral recumbent position in an attempt to localize fluid when pleural effusions are present.[13]

Other x-ray films frequently taken include tomograms and laminagrams. These films allow viewing of structures that are normally concealed by other structures. Fluoroscopic examination of the chest may be done. This allows the radiologist to look for evidence of a tumor by observing the dynamic activity of the chest.[13]

Since these tests may be time-consuming and tiring for the patient, assurance that they are necessary should be given.

It should be mentioned that chest x-ray screening programs have been carried out in attempts to detect cancer in early stages in susceptible segments of the population. Several extensive surveys have all reached the conclusion that large-scale x-ray screening at 6-month intervals does not actually alter the mortality from lung cancer.[8]

Obtaining sputum specimens for cytologic study is an essential part of the diagnostic workup for lung cancer. As cancer cells are exfoliated by the tumor, they are expelled in the sputum and are recognizable by their abnormal morphology when studied under the microscope.[13]

These specimens are best obtained early in the morning, since secretions tend to collect in the lungs while the patient sleeps. Sputum specimens are usually collected every morning for at least 3 days, since these cells may only be expelled intermittently. The specimen should be coughed directly into a container with a preservative solution in order to maintain the cell morphology.[13]

It is important that the patient cough deeply, producing a specimen from the bronchi, and that he not brush his teeth or use an antiseptic mouthwash before producing the specimen. Patients who cannot produce sputum may need a heated aerosol treatment to help stimulate production of secretions.[6]

Cytologic examinations are also done on fluid aspirated from a pleural effusion. The presence of malignant cells in pleural fluid often contraindicates surgery, since the tumor may be disseminated rapidly via the lymph vessels to other parts of the body.[13]

Bronchoscopy is a procedure used to aid in diagnosing lung tumors by allowing the physician to examine the interior of the bronchial tree. This examination gives the surgeon clues regarding the nature of the lesion and its extension to adjacent structures. It may indicate whether or not the lesion is resectable. Even if the lesion is not visible during bronchoscopy, bronchial washings may aid in cytologic diagnosis.

In recent years a flexible fiberoptic bronchoscope has replaced the rigid tube that was formerly used for this examination. Fiberoptic materials redirect light and transmit it around numerous twists and bends. This type of bronchoscope allows for visualization of the segmental bronchi and their bifurcations, which could not be done with the rigid metal scopes. In addition, the conscious patient is more comfortable when this type of equipment is used, and the chances of endotracheal perforation are nearly nonexistent.[7]

Prior to the examination the patient is given nothing by mouth for 8 hours; a sedative is usually administered within an hour before the procedure. Bronchoscopy is usually done under local anesthesia, but general anesthesia may be used. It is performed in a darkened room, and the patient will be lying supine, with the head hyperextended and the eyes covered.[13]

After the examination is completed, the patient may resume eating only after the anesthesia is gone and the gag reflex returns, usually in 2 to 6 hours. Mild analgesics and warm saline gargles may relieve the discomfort in the throat caused by the tube. The patient should be observed for any signs of bleeding or respiratory distress. Sputum should be collected after the bronchoscopy, since passing the bronchoscope into the bronchial tree may cause some of the cancer cells to become dislodged.[13]

Whereas bronchoscopy is used to examine the larger bronchi, bronchography is a procedure for exploring the smaller bronchi for indications of disease. This examination is carried out by passing a small catheter into the bronchi either by way of the mouth or nose or through a tube passed directly into the trachea by means of a percutaneous stick. An opaque medium is then instilled through the tube. The patient is asked to assume various positions as different bronchi are studied under fluoroscopy.[13]

A brush biopsy may be done during bronchography by passing a small brush through the catheter. The tissue obtained by brushing the lesion is then sent for cytologic study.[2]

Preoperative and postoperative routines for bronchography are the same as for bronchoscopy. In addition, the patient is instructed to place his finger over the puncture site if a needle was passed into the trachea to prevent subcutaneous emphysema.

Tissue biopsies may also be taken from different sites in diagnosing lung carcinomas. Scalene and mediastinal lymph nodes are biopsied to determine whether metastasis has occurred whenever (1) the nodes are palpable; (2) the tumor is large or of known long duration; or (3) oat cell carcinoma is suspected.[13]

Biopsies of the pleura may be done during a routine thoracocentesis with a special biopsy needle. Tissue from a suspected lesion may be obtained either by percutaneous aspiration through a needle under fluoroscopy or surgically through a small thoracotomy incision.

In patients being considered for thoracic surgery, pulmonary function tests are usually done. Some patients who have tumors that are possibly resectable are not candidates for a thoracotomy because of significant impairment of lung function due to other types of pulmonary diseases. The pulmonary function tests include complete lung function studies and resting and arterial blood gas determinations.[3]

The patient may also undergo diagnostic examination, such as brain or bone scans, to determine whether the cancer has spread to distant organs.

SURGICAL THERAPY

In evaluating patients for thoracic surgery, the physician contemplates several things. The growth pattern of the particular type of cancer that has been diagnosed and the probable response of the type to the various forms of therapy available are important considerations. An oat cell carcinoma that grows and spreads rapidly is usually considered inoperable but responds dramatically to radiation therapy and chemotherapy, although this response is generally short-lived. Adenocarcinomas and squamous cell lesions have a better chance of being removed surgically.[13]

The extent of the cancer at the time of therapy is also considered. Metastasis to extrathoracic regions, to lymph nodes, to the opposite lung, or to the parietal pleura renders the cancer unresectable. Involvement of the phrenic nerve, the recurrent laryngeal nerve, or the pulmonary artery, and signs of superior vena cava obstruction are also criteria for inoperability.[4,13] The ability of the patient to withstand the surgery must be taken into consideration. Cardiac, hepatic, and other pulmonary diseases often contraindicate surgery.

Also considered will be the patient's age and what Hinshaw[4] refers to as "the skilled physician's estimate of the vague factor of a tenacious hold upon life, which defies description but is nonetheless real and often of considerable importance."

If a person is considered to be a surgical candidate, he is taken to the operating room for an exploratory thoracotomy. If it is evident that the tumor cannot be entirely removed, a pulmonary resection is not usually performed. It was at one time thought that the primary tumor should be removed for palliative reasons. Instead it has been demonstrated that life expectancy and comfort of the patient have been decreased by this procedure.[13]

When the tumor can be removed in its entirety, only that portion of the lung which is involved will be resected. A lobectomy, the removal of one lobe of the lung, may be adequate for total resection of the tumor. This procedure is preferred to conserve more functional lung tissue. A pneumonectomy, the removal of one whole lung, is generally performed only when a cancer has invaded the main bronchus of a lung to such a degree that there are no alternatives.[13]

The patient must be taught before surgery what to expect postoperatively so that there will be no undue fright because of the routines and equipment.

Postoperatively, meticulous pulmonary therapy is paramount in order to prevent further compromise of the lung function. This includes encouraging the patient to cough, giving nasotracheal suctioning as needed, turning the patient at frequent intervals, and ambulating as soon as possible. After a pneumonectomy, the patient should be only partially turned to either side. Some surgeons prefer that the patient be turned only to the operative side. These precautions prevent mediastinal shift and compression of the remaining lung.[6]

Chest tubes are used to obtain a negative pressure in the chest by allowing air and fluid to drain out of the pleural space and enabling the lung to reexpand postoperatively. Pneumonectomy patients generally do not have chest tubes, since it is desirable for the empty thoracic space to fill with serous exudate, which eventually consolidates and aids in preventing mediastinal shift.[6]

The patient must be observed for such postoperative complications as bleeding, mediastinal shift, airway obstruction, pulmonary edema and emboli, and respiratory insufficiency.

For a guide to the complete management of the thoracic surgery patient, see Luckmann and Sorensen.[6]

RADIATION THERAPY AND CHEMOTHERAPY
FOR LUNG CANCER PATIENTS

For those persons in whom the tumor is found to be unresectable, radiotherapy, chemotherapy, or both may be instigated. These measures may bring the patient some temporary relief of exasperating symptoms such as pain, cough, or hemoptysis, but a cure of the disease is quite unlikely.

Preoperative irradiation may be done occasionally to produce some regression of the tumor and to more clearly delineate it. Irradiation prior to surgery may also devitalize the cancer cells somewhat so that the risk of disseminating these cells through the bloodstream during surgery will be decreased.[13]

Extrathoracic structures such as the brain and bones may be irradiated to relieve neurologic symptoms and the severe pain of bone metastasis. Bone irradiation may also help to prevent pathologic fractures.

Side effects of radiation therapy are dependent on the area of the body that is being irradiated. Bone marrow depression and skin breakdown are common in these patients.

Several groups of drugs have been found to be helpful in providing some palliative effects in patients with lung cancer. They are chiefly the alkylating agents and antimetabolites. Experimental agents may also be used. For a summary of major antineoplastic drugs, side effects, and related nursing care, see the list in Chapter 6.

To control malignant pleural effusions, a sclerosing substance is often instilled into the pleural cavity through a chest tube. Nitrogen mustard preparations and quinacrine hydrochloride (Atabrine) are the drugs commonly used for this purpose. The patient may experience fever, nausea, and bone marrow depression after this therapy.[9]

The patient whose cancer is found to be inoperable and who begins radiation treatments or chemotherapy often begins to realize at this time that the condition is incurable. It is important for the nurse to spend a great deal of time in answering questions about the treatment and exploring fears that may be expressed.

The patient's general condition should be maintained during the therapy. This is often difficult as the side effects of nausea and vomiting, anorexia, mouth lesions, and bone marrow depression occur. It is sometimes helpful to administer antiemetics prior to meals or as needed to control nausea and vomiting. Scheduling of treatments so that they are not given close to mealtime is helpful. Topical anesthetics and a soft or liquid diet may be necessary for patients with ulcerations of the mouth. Sufficient rest should be provided, since the treatments may result in weakness. Mild tranquilizers or sedatives may be beneficial.

These patients should have blood tests, including frequent white blood cell counts, differential counts, platelet counts, and hemoglobin determinations. If the patient's white blood cell count is diminishing, it becomes exceedingly important that the nursing staff and the patient practice strict hygienic measures. The patient should avoid contact with persons with infectious diseases, and good oral hygiene must be emphasized.

Fluids must be forced, to keep the patient well hydrated when medications that can cause hemorrhagic cystitis are being used. Testing the urine for occult blood may be initiated by the nursing staff. Prior to hematuria the patient may experience urinary frequency and dysuria for several days. Administering drugs that produce this side effect early in the day will help to prevent the toxic metabolic end products from accumulating in the bladder during the night.[10]

The patient should be taught how to care for the skin over the irradiated area. If irritation of the skin occurs, special ointments may be prescribed by the radiologist, but the use of soap and water, powder, alcohol, or heating pads is contraindicated.[13]

Esophagitis or tracheobronchitis may need to be treated if they occur as the result of the radiation therapy and are a discomfort to the patient.

Radiation therapy may be carried out over a period of 3 to 8 weeks. Patients may receive fifteen or more courses of chemotherapy, with the treatments being given 6 weeks apart. Consequently, these patients may be cared for at home. It is important to determine before discharge what activities the patient can accomplish and who will be available to help with the other tasks. Nursing or convalescent home placement or a referral to a public health or visiting nurse agency may be necessary.

GUIDELINES FOR NURSING CARE
OF LUNG CANCER PATIENTS

If nursing intervention is to be beneficial, certain guidelines must be taken into consideration when assessing the patient and planning care.

In educating persons about the hazards of smoking and air pollution, the nurse must keep in mind that persons are not likely to change their life-styles and take action unless they believe that they are susceptible to cancer and that it may have a very serious effect on their lives. Persons must also be aware of specific measures that can be taken to prevent cancer. The nurse will need to make suggestions as to how the individual can stop smoking, such as attending smoking withdrawal clinics and joining certain groups who are interested in the problem.

The nursing assessment of the patient who enters the hospital for a diagnostic examination for suspected lung cancer should include specific information such as (1) risk factors that predispose the patient to the development of lung cancer; (2) status of the respiratory system; (3) the patient's understanding of the illness, feelings about it, and ability to cope with it; and (4) significant persons in the patient's life who will be present during hospitalization.

In a determination of the risk factors, the patient's occupation should be noted, since it may increase susceptibility to cancer of the lung. In addition, whether or not the patient smokes should be noted, and if so, how much and for how long.

The patient should also be asked about previous diagnoses or treatment of tumors in any other part of the body.

An assessment of the patient's respiratory system may also be made by the nurse. It is important to provide this baseline of information so that the patient's response to therapy can be better evaluated. A preoperative examination of the patient's respiratory status will also help the nurse to plan more effective postoperative interventions for the patient who is undergoing surgical diagnosis and treatment. A guide for assessing the thorax and lungs is given by Traver.[12]

Patients and their families need to be taught about the illness and about the diagnostic and therapeutic measures that will be taken, but before such teaching can be effective, the nurse must assess the patient's understanding of the illness and his feelings about it.

Fears and anxieties must also be explored. Many patients entering with one or more of the symptoms of lung cancer are particularly apprehensive about the effect that the cancer will eventually have on their ability to breathe. They are fearful that they will not be able to breathe during procedures when tubes and wires are advanced down their windpipes into their lungs.

Patients who enter without any symptoms other than a suspicious chest x-ray examination or sputum analysis may not consider themselves ill and may continue to deny their illness even after a positive diagnosis is made. Even patients presenting with symptoms such as a cough or hemoptysis who are discovered to have lung cancer may continue to deny the reality of the illness for some time.

Patients who are denying their illness often suppress and distort the information given to them. Explanations regarding the hospital setting and the diagnostic and therapeutic routines must be simple.

Patients sometimes become angry with those who try to force them to learn more about their illness while they are still incapable of accepting the diagnosis.

The patient who begins to ask questions about how the body functions and about the disease is usually ready to be taught more about the diagnosis, treatment, and prognosis.[5]

The preoperative period is often a particularly anxious time for the patient. There may be vacillation between the hope that the cancer can be completely resected and the fear that the tumor will have advanced beyond the reach of surgical extirpation. The staff needs to be aware of what the physician has told the patient regarding the results of the diagnostic tests and the prognosis of the disease.

Since the rate of cure for lung cancer is only 10%, the nurse will need to be able to aid the patient who is dying.

The nurse must also determine and assess the support mechanisms available to the patient, as well as identify the persons in the patient's life who are important and who will provide emotional support during the illness. The family's perception of the patient's illness and their expectations of the therapy must be assessed. Many times the patient's and the family's wishes differ in regard to how vigorous the therapy should be if the patient is found to be incurable.

The nurse should make available the information gained from the patient on the Kardex, the chart, or both. The nurse needs to recognize problems that are beyond the scope of nursing and to elicit the aid of other disciplines when necessary.

The patient may reenter the hospital on numerous occasions during the illness for further treatment. Therefore the nurse should summarize on discharge the nursing assessments made during the patient's hospitalization, the problems identified, the nursing intervention utilized, and the status of the problems at the time of discharge.

Mr. T. is an example of a patient hospitalized for a chest evaluation. He was a 55-year-old German immigrant baker. On admission a nursing history was obtained, and it revealed that Mr. T. had suffered from chronic obstructive lung disease for the previous 10 years. Prior to the development of lung disease he had smoked one and a half packs of cigarettes a day for 25 years. Mr. T. stated that since the time he began suffering from obstructive lung disease, he had had a chronic cough productive of yellow sputum. He consulted his family physician when he noted that for 2 weeks his cough had become more productive and the sputum had changed to a greenish color and was at times blood-tinged. Mr. T. also said that he was becoming increasingly short of breath and was having chills and fever. He mentioned that he seemed to have "a bad cold that he could not shake." Mr. T.'s doctor felt that a thorough chest workup was necessary.

Significant findings of the physical examination of the chest were coarse bibasilar rales and diffuse expiratory wheezes.

Mr. T.'s wife was present at the time of admission and stated that she would be with the patient most of the time while he was hospitalized. Both the patient and his wife appeared quite anxious and upset. They seemed to have some difficulty communicating in English, but they did express understanding and appreciation when the nurse spent much time explaining routines and procedures to them that were to be carried out in the hospital.

Sputum specimens were obtained and sent to the laboratory for culture, acid-fast bacilli, and cytology. The cytology and AFB (acid-fast bacilli) tests were negative, but the culture revealed that Mr. T. did have an infection, probably due to secretions trapped beyond a partially obstructed bronchus.

Tomograms of the chest revealed a nodule in the left upper lobe. A bronchoscopy was then done, the tumor was visualized, and adenocarcinoma cells were found in the bronchial washings.

Pulmonary function studies were carried out, and it was determined that surgery could not be offered to the patient, since he could not tolerate the loss of a lobe of his lung because of the preexisting lung disease.

It was decided to treat Mr. T. with radiation therapy on an outpatient basis.

After learning of his diagnosis and the treatment to be pursued, Mr. T. and his wife became quite despondent, communicating very little with any of the nursing or medical staff.

Since the patient was to be discharged soon, a public health nurse was asked to follow Mr. T. throughout his course of radiation therapy. This was considered necessary because it was believed that the patient needed further explanation of his disease and treatment, monitoring for complications of the therapy, and support as he began to realize the implications of his illness on his life.

SUMMARY

Lung cancer can be a particularly frightening and distressing disease for patients. Nursing intervention can be beneficial to the patient if a thorough nursing assessment is done, and care is planned with the individual patient in mind. A major responsibility of nurses lies in educating the public regarding prevention of lung cancer.

REFERENCES

1. Andrews, C. E.: Bronchogenic carcinoma. In Baum, G. L., editor: Textbook of pulmonary diseases, Boston, 1965, Little, Brown & Co.
2. Deeley, T. J.: Modern radiotherapy: carcinoma of the bronchus, New York, 1971, Appleton-Century-Crofts.
3. Gracey, D. R.: Preoperative pulmonary function evaluation, Heart and Lung **3:**500, May-June, 1971.
4. Hinshaw, H. C.: Diseases of the chest, Philadelphia, 1969, W. B. Saunders Co.
5. Lederer, H. D.: How the sick view their world. In Skipper, J. K., and Leonard, R. C., editors: Social interaction and patient care, Philadelphia, 1965, J. B. Lippincott Co.
6. Luckmann, J., and Sorensen, K. C.: Medical-surgical nursing, a psychophysiologic approach, Philadelphia, 1974, W. B. Saunders Co.
7. Marici, J. N.: The flexible fiberoptic bronchoscope, The American Journal of Nursing **73:**1776, Oct., 1973.

8. Rhodes, M. L., and others: Early detection of lung cancer, Chest **64:**741, Dec., 1973.
9. Rosenfeld, M. G.: Manual of therapeutics, Boston, 1971, Little, Brown & Co.
10. Schumann, D., and Patterson, P.: Multiple myeloma, The American Journal of Nursing **75:**78, Jan., 1975.
11. Stewart, M. S.: Cigarettes: American's No. 1 Health Problem, pamphlet no. 439A, New York, 1972, Public Affairs Committee.
12. Traver, G. A.: Assessment of the thorax and lungs, The American Journal of Nursing **73:**466, March, 1973.
13. Watson, W., editor: Lung cancer, St. Louis, 1968, The C. V. Mosby Co.

part IV
MAXIMIZING THE QUALITY OF LIFE

The valuable information and philosophies shared in the chapters in this part are the essence of cancer nursing. The theme running throughout the book, in fact, is a concern for the quality of life as well as the quality of care. Without this concern, our intervention for the cancer patient is reduced to that of a technician. These chapters imply that we have confronted our own feelings about cancer and that our reasons for choosing this field have been explored.

Again, the personal and patient experiences make these chapters unique and invaluable. They demonstrate the reward and beauty in sensitive and caring nursing. They incorporate techniques of crisis intervention along with support of the patients' and families' rights. How great it would be if each dying patient were given open communication, freedom from pain, and the choice of a place to die. These reachable goals are discussed in the following chapters.

12 Metastatic carcinoma of the breast

a comparison of its influence on the functional capacity of two women

VICKI ELIZABETH LONG

This chapter presents 2 female patients with metastatic carcinoma of the breast in the terminal phase of the disease. Although the course of the disease in these individuals is unique to this form of malignancy, the prescribed therapies, and the patients' respective personalities, in many ways they share similarities with all persons with malignancies. However, this chapter attempts to show, in a discussion of the classic description of metastatic carcinoma of the breast in relation to functional capacities of body systems and in comparison of 2 patients, that medical and nursing personnel should not allow these classic facts to stand in the way of caring for the whole human being. Rather, these generalizations should be used as a basis for coming to terms with the complexities of the disease and its individual manifestation in each patient's microenvironment.

In discussing the relationship of malignant neoplasms to body systems, one must consider as well the effect of specific therapies on these systems. As the disease increases in severity and treatment becomes progressively more radical, the side effects of therapy as well as the natural disease process become of major concern to nursing and medicine. In fact, it can almost be said that malignant neoplasms have no natural process in man because of the ability of modern western medical therapy to prolong life. The natural course of a malignancy is a disruption or breakdown of homeostasis and eventual cessation of bodily functions. Medical treatment alters and often distorts homeostatic mechanisms in its attempt to slow down the disruptive malignant processes. It is my opinion that the great breakthrough in medicine has not been the eradication of some malignancies nor even the easing of pain associated with these malignancies but rather the prolonging of life so that the affected individual receives the opportunity to come to terms with death. Thus the balance between the agony of the disease and its treatment and the will to live in patients with malignancy is a fine one.

The functions of the body are discussed in thirteen categories as presented by Mitchell[10]: psychosocial status, mental and emotional status, environmental status, sensory status, motor status, nutritional status, elimination status, circulatory status,

149

respiratory status, temperature status, fluid and electrolyte status, integumentary status, and comfort and rest status. In discussing these categories in relation to the 2 patients presented, it is assumed that the reader accepts that the following information has been gathered during assessment, the first component of the nursing process. Problem identification, goal definition, action proposal, action implementation, action evaluation, and action modification are the remaining steps of that process.

The following discussion of the influence of metastatic carcinoma of the breast on the functional capacity of Anne and Sybil (the names have been changed) focuses on problems that concerned nursing personnel during a 3-day period in the terminal phase of the illness. Information pertinent to nursing responsibility when a patient is in a preterminal condition is included in the area of mental and emotional status, since this area readily affects all patients, regardless of prognosis. Where possible, data on medical therapy, consultations, and laboratory studies are included as necessary considerations for ongoing assessment.

PSYCHOSOCIAL STATUS

Assessment of psychosocial status is an important nursing function. It begins with a well-documented patient history, which is continually updated by individuals participating in patient care. Through interviews with the patient and significant others, one can establish a picture of family network systems, financial and social status, and educational background, as well as medical facts. Statistical data relevant to the particular disease process should be reviewed at this time, with attention to their significance in relation to the patient concerned. This is a realistic way to establish support systems for each patient while developing individualized nursing plans for care.

Breast cancer is the most common malignancy in women, the leading cause of malignant death in females, and, in the premenopausal period, the leading cause of death in women. It occurs quite often in young women but most often immediately precedes or follows menopause. Studies have shown a higher incidence in single women, women who are childless and have a familial history of carcinoma of the breast.[13] Sex itself is a factor, since breast carcinoma is rare in males.[2] The World Health Organization reports that the woman is at a disadvantage because endogenous estrogens have a depressant action on bone marrow, which increases the chance of complications due to anemia resulting from therapy and disease.[1]

Anne was a 50-year-old white woman, married and with no children. She was at the 5-year mark in the course of her illness. Details of her medical therapy include the following:

Year 1: Right radical mastectomy with positive axillary node involvement, followed by two courses of cobalt treatment.
Year 2: Remission supposed.
Year 3: Malignant left pleural effusion diagnosis.
Year 4: Left pleural effusion with metastases to ninth rib with streptococcal pneumonia

after laparoscopy revealing abdominal metastases. Palliative salpingectomy, oophorectomy, and bilateral adrenalectomy performed. Chemotherapy begun.

Year 5: Possible Addisonian crisis due to poor maintenance of steroids.
Aspiration of vomitus, possible pneumonia.
Fever (103° F.) and gastrointestinal distress.

Sybil was a 41-year-old white woman, married, with 3 children. She, too, was at the fifth year of illness. Details of her medical therapy include the following:

Year 1: Modified left mastectomy for infiltrating ductal carcinoma with no lymph node involvement.

Year 2: Temporary remission.

Year 3: Fluoride scan revealed lesions in left femur; low lumbar spine involvement.

Year 4: Multiple skeletal involvement noted, with radiation to hip, spine, pelvis, and femur. Therapeutic salpingectomy, oophorectomy, and bilateral adrenalectomy. Chemotherapy and androgen therapy begun.

Year 5: Increased spinal involvement with radiation to the third lumber and occipital regions.
Fever (102° F.), gastrointestinal distress, and increased pain.

Anne's and Sybil's cases support epidemiologic data associated with a classic definition of carcinoma of the breast. Both followed similar courses of therapy. Although their areas of metastases differed, abdominal and skeletal sites are both common.[2]

MENTAL AND EMOTIONAL STATUS

A diagnosis of carcinoma of the breast is a challenge to both patient and health professional because of the significance of the breast to cultural roles. The fear of death is augmented by the fear of physical mutilation of surgical mastectomy. Weisman[14] states that victims of malignancy may have more reason to deny than other terminally ill patients but because of "insistent, refractory symptoms" have less chance to do so. Considering the constant reminder of ones diagnosis after mastectomy, the sufferer of carcinoma of the breast would have even less chance to forget her illness.

Yet, denial plagues us in the face of the reality of cancer as a possibility, for malignancy exists for us all. There are four general areas in which nursing comes face to face with denial and carcinoma of the breast. The first is in the area of prevention: a woman needs to understand that although the possibility of malignancy does exist, early detection and treatment increase the chance of survival (Chapter 4). Second is the preparation for a surgical procedure either to aid in diagnosis or arrest malignancy. Third is the area of living as full a life as possible postoperatively, and fourth is the most relevant to this chapter: acceptance of a terminal illness.

The area of mental and emotional status concerns the consequences of hormonal imbalance that may occur as a result of therapy. Alterations in hormonal balance may result from removal of all or part of the reproductive system, adrenalectomy with subsequent steroid maintenance, hypophysectomy, the cessation of post-menopausal estrogen therapy, or treatment with androgens.[1]

Anne and Sybil received systemic administration of the glucocorticoids predni-solone and fludrocortisone (Florinef) because of bilateral adrenalectomy. Sub-jectively it was noted that Anne handled anxiety less effectively than did Sybil. Anne was described as a perfectionist by the staff, one who was compulsively or-ganized, whereas Sybil was known to be more tolerant of disorganization. Anne's order for steroids included conditions to increase her dosage when stress became obvious. Although both Anne and Sybil were from the same socioeconomic back-ground and had both held professional positions, Sybil chose to work until patho-logic fractures immobilized her. Anne ceased working soon after diagnosis, which is perhaps another indication of how she tolerated stress.

ENVIRONMENTAL STATUS

As mentioned previously, adrenalectomy calls for a decrease in the level of stress offered by one's environment, especially while steroid therapy is being instigated. Chemotherapy causes concern for infection control, since depressed immune response is a side effect of this course of therapy.[12] Protective isolation may be required. Safety after mastectomy may be a problem because the ability to maintain normal balance may be affected due to a change in the body's center of gravity.[13] It is therefore necessary that the room be as conveniently arranged and as free of hazards as possible during the immediate postoperative period. Potential skeletal involvement with metastatic lesions, resulting in weakened, de-mineralized bone, calls for protective measures such as raising of side rails, in-stalling an overhead trapeze, and initiating other measures to make motion safe.

Anne and Sybil presented different problems that called for protective measures. On her last admission, Anne showed a white blood count depressed to 250 cells/cu. mm.; Protective isolation measures were instigated. Due to gastrointestinal upset as a consequence of chemotherapy and abdominal metastases, she was maintained on intravenous fluids. Because of her feverish state, these intravenous sites called for protective measures to minimize trauma. Bed rest was ordered. Bed rest was a necessity for Sybil as well. Her pathologic fractures from skeletal metastases de-manded that safety rails be raised at all times and that a trapeze be used, with no weight bearing allowed. Although her white blood count was depressed to 3,900 cells/cu. mm., protective isolation was not felt to be necessary.

SENSORY STATUS

Heightened sensitivity to pain is the primary issue in the area of sensory status. Metastasis plays a role in increased pain, since the areas affected are often more vascular and have greater innervation or body function than the primary site. Recall that lungs, liver, bones, and the gastrointestinal system are common sites for metastases in carcinoma of the breast.[2] Spinal metastases may cause variations in sensation and an inability to respond in a normal fashion to intact nerves.[2] One must also consider alterations in diet because of abdominal involvement or as a result of therapy, of decreasing taste sensation, and of decreasing desire for food intake. However, since intractable pain is associated with malignancy,[14] this aspect of sensory status will be paramount.

Similarities between Anne and Sybil vanished in considering alterations in sensory status. Anne was on a liquid diet and was experiencing much anorexia, and the decreased sensation of taste further inhibited her appetite. Her general sensory input was decreased due to protective isolation, but since her pain was insignificant, she was able to enjoy listening to the radio and reading. Sybil, however, was experiencing extreme pain that interfered with her ability to receive input. Her pain often reached the point of delirium. She was to receive "pain cocktail" every 4 hours as needed. It consisted of methadone (a narcotic analgesic), 10 mg. in 5 ml. of syrup, followed by 5 mg. of the tranquilizer Valium orally, which she requested regularly. She enjoyed the taste of food immensely and remarked that this was one of the few things she could enjoy, since being flat on her back made other input difficult. However, since nausea interfered with her ability to enjoy this one positive input, an antiemetic was ordered.

MOTOR STATUS

Patients who have had a mastectomy and consequent alteration of the center of gravity need help in regaining stability. Edema associated with lymph node removal may decrease mobility due to protective immobility. However, the potential for skeletal metastasis is of prime concern in relation to motor status. Every effort must be made to avoid the complications of immobility resulting from skeletal involvement, including decubiti, increased work load to the heart, and decreased respiratory capacity.[10]

Sybil fit the classic description of the patient immobilized by skeletal metastases and pain. Weight bearing was impossible, and she had been unable to tolerate the head of her bed raised. Anne's mobility was restricted by administration of intravenous fluid and by the limited horizon of protective isolation. Her general debilitation due to gastrointestinal upset and anorexia caused much weakness and made all movement tiring.

NUTRITIONAL STATUS

The nutritional status of a patient suffering from a malignancy is one of the primary concerns of total care in the battle to maintain homeostasis. *The Nursing Mirror and Midwives Journal* devoted a series of three articles to the subject of nutrition and malignancy in 1972. It points to the increased metabolic demands due to malignancy,[4] the general loss of well-being and anorexia that may come from worry and anxiety due to the diagnosis,[3] and the complications for the gastrointestinal system due to therapy.[5] Generally, increasing catabolism that cannot be rectified seems to be a primary concern.

Specific alterations in carbohydrate metabolism, protein metabolism, and lipid metabolism are discussed in detail by Hoch-Ligeti[8] and are beyond the scope of this chapter. However, generally speaking, alterations in carbohydrate metabolism may involve hypoglycemia and hyperglycemia, protein swing is usually to negative nitrogen balance that cannot be replaced, and fat metabolism varies greatly with the area of metastasis.[8] Anne's anorexia and increase in nausea and vomiting greatly interfered with her ability to tolerate solid foods. She was maintained on oral bland liquids served at room temperature, with supplemental intravenous fluids of D_5W alternated with D_5 and 0.5N saline solution. Sybil, however, was encouraged to eat solid foods when she could tolerate them. Her inability to ingest was directly related to gastrointestinal complications of chemotherapy and radiation. Anne suffered the consequences of chemotherapy as well, but it can be assumed that her abdominal metastasis will cause permanent alterations in diet. A previous liver scan noted possible metastasis to that organ, with further disrupted metabolism expected.

ELIMINATION STATUS

Elimination systems, both bowel and bladder, may be affected by obstruction or metastasis. Specific malignancy therapies that affect the gastrointestinal system alter elimination as well as nutrition. When skeletal metastases are a consideration, sphincter control becomes a concern. Difficulty in micturition is common.[2] A close watch must be kept for loss of control, care must be taken to avoid further trauma to the spincters, and rehabilitation should be instigated when possible. Adrenalectomy necessitates medical therapy to compensate for the loss of all adrenal hormones, catecholamines, glucocorticoids and mineral corticoids, with compensation for the loss of aldosterone, which causes alterations in elimination. Severe nephropathy has also been reported in patients on chemotherapy.[12]

Regions of metastasis influenced elimination status for Anne and Sybil. Anne's gastrointestinal involvement and bland diet, coupled with chemotherapy, made diarrhea a problem, and occult blood was noticed in her stools. Sybil suffered diarrhea as a consequence of chemotherapy and radiation, but as yet she had not had difficulty with micturition. Positioning made the act of elimination very difficult for Sybil, however.

CIRCULATORY, RESPIRATORY, AND TEMPERATURE STATUS

These body systems are best considered together because of the interrelationships between respiration and circulation.

Circulation may be impaired by obstruction or may serve as a focus for metastatic spread. Circulation to the breast is extensive: blood flows to the breast tissue by way of the internal mammary arteries, the axillary arteries, and small tributaries of the intercostals. It is drained by a similarly extensive, corresponding venous system. Lymphatic drainage is also widespread. The extensive lymphatic system of this area includes the axillary nodes, the supraclavicular and infraclavicular nodes, and the internal mammary chain. In considering circulatory status, one must consider the threat of Addisonian crisis, which may be the result of inadequate adrenal functioning or insufficient replacement steroids. Hypotension and total circulatory collapse may occur, resulting in coma and death.[13]

Increase in temperature usually is present in individuals suffering from malignancy, but the etiology is unknown. It may be a sign of secondary systemic infection caused by the decreased immune response associated with chemotherapy. Persistent fever in lieu of general increased metabolism may be noticed.

Effusions and lung involvement, which are possibilities with carcinoma of the breast, result in decreased respiratory capacity. Confinement to bed may compromise respiratory mechanisms, as would skeletal metastasis to the ribs. According to Dickerson: "It seems clear that the activity of neoplastic disease requires a greater than normal expenditure of energy, which is derived initially from a breakdown of body fat. Patients with cancer therefore have a low respiratory quotient."[3] Furthermore, with carcinoma of the breast one must consider the alterations of the chest wall with mastectomy, the removal of muscles from that area, and the possibility of interference with innervation to the intercostal muscles, which may interfere with respiration.

Anne and Sybil both exhibited alterations in temperature due to the effects of chemotherapy. Anne's pulse was constantly elevated to 110 and was weak and thready. Sybil's pulse rose with her delirium from pain to 112. Both had orders to notify their physicians should the pulse rate increase to 140. This increase may be assumed to be related to failure of steroid maintenance to compensate for loss of the adrenal gland, making an increased dosage in steroid replacement mandatory. Anne's laboratory values showed evidence of saline depletion, but she did not exhibit clinical alterations in blood pressure. Respiratory capacity for both patients was clinically normal. However, Anne's lung secretions were increased because of possible aspiration pneumonia, making respiration a concern. Oxygen was available for both patients in case of emergency.

FLUID AND ELECTROLYTE STATUS

Disturbances of the gastrointestinal tract as well as increased metabolism point to potential fluid and electrolyte imbalance. All routine laboratory values may show alteration. Some that are specific in the patient with malignancy of the breast include hyponatremia due to therapeutic adrenalectomy, and subsequent loss of aldosterone with the failure of replacement therapy to adequately supply this important mineral corticoid. A further complication is the therapeutic addition of androgens, which may, because no pure androgen has yet been manufactured, contain some aldosterone. This addition may lead to hypernatremia if androgens and steroids are combined. Hypercalcemia, associated with bone involvement and increased osteoclast activity, may occur with or without skeletal metastasis.[8] Potassium imbalances may occur with extreme alterations in gastrointestinal and kidney function.[6]

Irradiation and chemotherapy must be generally considered as potential sources of electrolyte and fluid imbalance, primarily due to gastrointestinal upset.[11] Because antineoplastic drugs have an increased effect on rapidly proliferating tissue, one must consider as well their specific alteration of gastrointestinal and oral mucosa.[12] This alteration could cause long-range problems in electrolyte imbalance even though gastrointestinal distress may stabilize with adaptation. Renal failure has also been reported with the administration of the antineoplastic agent methotrexate,[12] necessitating large amounts of fluids, which may cause difficulties for a patient unable to tolerate oral fluids. Obviously, the complicated relationship between the need for increased fluids and therapeutic diet alterations, as well as metabolic shifts, makes electrolyte monitoring a must.

The gastrointestinal upset experienced by Anne and Sybil necessitated saline replacement. However, intravenous administration of saline solution did not alleviate Anne's saline depletion. Potassium levels for both patients remained within normal limits, but careful monitoring continued due to constant alterations in gastrointestinal function and possible consequences of alterations in aldosterone. Interestingly, Sybil did not show a serum calcium inbalance, despite significant skeletal metastasis. Due to chemotherapy, both patients received increased fluids orally as tolerated, and intravenously when necessary, to prevent renal complications.

INTEGUMENTARY STATUS

Most alterations in the integument are due to essential shifts in metabolism, with potential decrease in protein intake as well as increased catabolism and electrolyte imbalance, resulting in a decrease in the general health of the integument. One must consider the therapies for malignancy to be contributing factors in the alteration of the integument. Bronzing of the skin may be associated with cushingoid symptoms after steroid replacement with adrenalectomy. The skin may darken in fields of irradition. An overall drying of the skin and loss of hair may occur with this course of treatment as well. Ulcer and fistula formation may eventually cause radiation treatment to be discontinued.

Chemotherapy produces radical alterations in integument.[7] Since hair follicles are rapidly proliferating tissues and therefore subject to the effects of cytotoxic drugs, loss of hair can be expected. Many varieties of dermatologic reactions have been reported after chemotherapy, including erythematous rashes, pruritus, urticaria, petechiae, ecchymoses, and photosensitivity.[12]

Integument problems occurring in both Anne and Sybil were related to specific therapies. Anne showed a great amount of hair loss daily after chemotherapy, which was distressing to her. There was no obvious darkening of her skin from radiation, nor did she have dermatologic signs of steroid replacement. Her skin was extremely pale and dry. Sybil, on the other hand, exhibited darkening of skin at joints from radiation therapy and a general bronzing of the skin from steroids. She had a characteristic cushingoid face. Her skin turgor was good, and there were no dermatologic signs of complications of immobility. Her hair was intact, with the exception of a patch in the occipital region from radiation.

COMFORT AND REST STATUS

The importance of comfort and rest in the patient with carcinoma of the breast cannot be overemphasized. In all patients with a malignancy, the increase in metabolic needs leads to increased requirements for rest in the body's fight to establish homeostasis disrupted by interference with all body systems due to the pathophysiology of the disease. As has been mentioned, pain associated with cancer is often intractable. The high doses of narcotics common in terminal stages of a malignancy are often not sufficient to provide comfort.

Decreases in sensory input are often necessary, since the alterations in rest patterns due to hospitalization and increased activity of tests and therapy may drain emotional resources. It should be emphasized that although therapies may seem passive to the patient, they involve extreme internal work that drains physiologic resources. As has been emphasized throughout this chapter, therapies may cause pain. Just as there will always be some need for varying degrees of pain intervention, there will always be a need to help the patient find satisfaction and comfort by making treatment and activities of daily living as restful as possible, while still allowing the affected individual the right to participate in self-care.

For Anne and Sybil, status of comfort and rest took on increased significance due to their progression toward death. Anne's reaction to stress made maintenance of a restful environment difficult. Sybil's increasing pain necessitated hydrotherapy, a quiet environment, and consistent administration of methadone (a narcotic analgesic) and diazepam (Valium) (a tranquilizer).

During the 3 days of care under discussion, several problems challenged nursing ingenuity. Formulating individual plans of care for Anne and Sybil involved identifying *current* difficulties based on assessment of present functional status, taking into account prescribed medical therapies. The underlying objective of recognizing problems for planning nursing care was to augment medical action in treating the person as well as the pathology.

Anne's problems, as delineated by the staff, were headed by gastrointestinal disturbances and were characterized by nausea, vomiting, and diarrhea. Such disturbances were secondary to metastases and recent chemotherapy. A severely depressed white blood count, high temperature, compromised respiratory capacity, and deterioration of integument were problems also resulting from disease process and therapies combined. Her anxiety and anger, thought to be due in part to difficulty in relinquishing control of her care to the staff, were major obstacles to comfort and rest.

Sybil's problems, although similar to Anne's, reflected the nature of the course her illness had taken. Pain from extensive bone metastases was the obvious primary problem. Fever, possibly resulting from chemotherapy, increased her discomfort. Immobility, with subsequent problems of respiratory function, transport safety, elimination, and integument integrity, was a major hurdle for patient and staff. Depression in the face of a hopeless prognosis and anxiety surrounding a proposed homecoming were also seen as priority problems.

Goals designed to diminish and, when feasible, eliminate these problems were defined. Major goals for Anne were as follows:

1. Prevention of fluid and electrolyte imbalance secondary to fever and gastrointestinal disturbances
2. Prevention of infection
3. Maintenance of respiratory function
4. Prevention of external trauma to integument
5. Decrease in anxiety
6. Understanding of source of hostility

Priority nursing goals established for Sybil were as follows:

1. Minimizing of pain secondary to bone metastases and prescribed therapies
2. Maintenance of respiratory capacity
3. Maintenance of intact integument
4. Provision for safety in transport
5. Expression of depression allowed
6. Decrease in anxiety in lieu of preparation for discharge

Actions proposed to meet these goals were derived from a synthesis of present functional capabilities and disabilities, keeping in mind the terminal state of Anne's and Sybil's disease processes. The success of nursing plans at this point involved more than implementing ideas—from on-the-spot evaluations, staff consultations, and honest confrontation with patients and significant others evolved action revisions. The following "conditions of an appropriate death" seemed a sensitive and positive base for directing modification of nursing actions in caring for Anne and Sybil: Someone who dies an appropriate death must be helped in the following ways. She should be relatively pain-free, her suffering reduced and emotional and social impoverishment kept to a minimum. Within the limits of disability, she should operate on as high and effective a level as possible, even though only tokens of former fulfillments can be offered. She should also recognize and resolve residual conflicts, and satisfy whatever remaining wishes are consistent with her present plight and with her ego ideal. Finally, among her choices, she should be able to yield control to others in whom she has confidence.*

Nursing actions specific for Anne's goals centered on providing necessary nourishment and fluids to combat the effects of gastrointestinal disturbances. Serving her full liquid diet at room temperature decreased stomach upset, but finding palatable substances was difficult. Dietary consultations including Anne and the hospital dietitian were planned. Individually blended cream vegetable soups be-

---

*Modified, with permission, from Weisman, A. D.: On dying and denying: a psychiatric study of terminality, New York, 1972, Behavioral Publications.

came her favorite selection. Small, frequent feedings were ordered. The staff cooperated by making mealtime as pleasant as possible. Her room was straightened before she was served, and she was helped to wash, complete oral care, and change her gown. Anne was offered an antiemetic, prochlorperazine maleate (Compazine), 10 mg intramuscularly (four times a day, as needed), approximately 20 minutes before major meals, but she rarely accepted the option. Anne did not enjoy conversation while eating, and since maintaining a stress-free environment was important, no other activities were planned surrounding her mealtime if possible.

To monitor her gastrointestinal disturbances, strict intake and output records were kept. All stools and vomitus were tested for occult blood with guaiac reagent. Electrolyte studies were reviewed as soon as they were processed by the laboratory.

Protective isolation, ordered because of Anne's severely depressed leukocyte count and increasing pleural effusion, aided in preventing infection and thereby maintaining respiratory capacity, but it hindered efficient interaction with the staff. To decrease stress and to increase Anne's confidence in the staff's ability to be organized in this situation, a virtue she obviously would value, we consulted her on her preference for arranging her personal effects and for communicating with staff members. We made it clear that we were open to suggestions.

When we learned that her family was accustomed to helping her with her bath and were knowledgeable concerning the importance of minimizing trauma to her integument, we planned this activity for a time when they would be present. They brought her favorite lotion from home. Their careful attention, the use of well-laundered cotton gowns and sheets, and the use of sheepskin pads in bed aided in retarding skin breakdown. We all encouraged Anne's wearing of wigs, and she was helped to apply makeup when she so desired.

Decreasing Anne's anxiety in the face of her desire to avoid discussion of her prognosis was a difficult task. Because she had undergone a bilateral adrenalectomy, it was necessary that her vital signs be used as a monitor of her stress level. The taking of vital signs became a constant reminder to Anne of her increasing anxiety. As the severity of symptoms increased, however, she was able to relinquish more control of her care to the staff. Our attention to the routine we now knew she preferred showed Anne our respect for her rights, and she began to rest more easily.

Perhaps the most difficult task faced was helping Anne to understand that the hostility she displayed was natural. The staff perceived her to be in what Kübler-Ross[9] calls the "anger state of dying." While we were most vulnerable, Anne's protective isolation served to "protect" us. The necessary gowns, gloves, and masks supplied barriers to touching and looking. We tried to overcome part of this problem by making a practice of turning to talk to Anne after we had unmasked at her door. She said that this action helped her to envision us while we were caring for her. Staff consultations on our feelings toward Anne helped us to vent our hostility toward her constant criticism. By learning to accept her criticisms without defensiveness and by showing her our willingness to provide her with care that took into consideration her feelings as well as ours, we were able to establish trust.

Nursing actions specific for Sybil centered on efforts to minimize the intractable pain she was experiencing primarily due to pathologic fractures. She regularly requested the "pain cocktail" that had been ordered every 4 hours as needed (10 mg. of the narcotic analgesic methadone in 5 ml. of syrup, followed by a tranquilizer, Valium, 5 mg. taken orally). As even slight movement added to her discomfort, activities of daily living were carefully timed after "pain cocktail" administration when drug action had peaked. She remained supine at all times, and we cut a small donut hole in a flat piece of foam rubber to accommodate the irradiated occipital site.

Hydrotherapy, which was ordered as a comfort measure, was discontinued at her request. She found the transfers to and from the stretcher and the ride back to her room on the then-wet canvas sling unbearable. We tried increasing the length of her bed baths at this point, using very warm water and gentle massage. Care was taken to avoid chilling and to adequately support her limbs. She remarked how much she enjoyed these baths, since they did more than increase her physical comfort: they provided her with soothing human touch and an opportunity for relaxed conversation.

Since skin care was of vital concern, her integument was regularly assessed during her bath. Lotion was used liberally, with gentle massage. An alternating airflow mattress helped to distribute pressure.

Sybil enjoyed her meals despite the transient nausea and vomiting resulting from chemotherapy. She regularly requested the antiemetic Compazine. Since she found food to be one of her few enjoyable sensations, the staff made sure that she received a variety of textures and temperatures. She needed help with feeding, and she appreciated an unhurried atmosphere. As well as the food itself, Sybil enjoyed the attention and social interaction surrounding her meals. When family members were present, they took over this task, but we often remained with them so that we could all enjoy Sybil during one of her favorite activities.

Immobility was a hurdle for all of us. We encouraged Sybil to cough to avoid stasis of respiratory secretions, but it was difficult because of spinal metastases. We kept side rails raised on her bed at all times, provided her with an overbed trapeze, and had at least three people present for every transfer. We aided her in use of the bedpan by supporting her back well with pillows during its use.

Aside from the time staff members spent with Sybil during pleasant tasks, time was allotted for just sitting with her. She was open about expressing her feelings concerning her imminent death and needed to be heard just as openly. She was often harsh with the staff, as was Anne, but we made efforts to let her know that we understood her frustration. Anxiety surrounded her proposed homecoming, partially from her fear of the increased pain involved with such a move and partially from her inability to curb her depression. We had to prepare her physically to return home, gradually raising the head of her bed until she could tolerate 30 minutes upright. Emotional preparation was equally important. We encouraged her to talk of the things she could experience only at home, letting her share with us stories of her children, pets, and favorite possessions. While we provided her with the best care possible, we helped her to realize that there were joys remaining to be experienced, perhaps for the last time.

A comparison of 2 patients with a similar diagnosis points to some valuable conclusions for nursing care of the patient with a malignancy. Perhaps the first is the value of a sound basis of knowledge when approaching a disease process in relation to individuals. An understanding of expected manifestations and underlying causes can be of assistance in pinpointing symptoms and compensating for distress that cannot be permanently alleviated. The second is the value of comparing patients with the same problems, which hopefully can lead to insights that facilitate the broadening of clinical judgment, increasing one's ability to discriminate between expected clinical signs and idiosyncratic behavior. A third conclusion gives impetus to the hypothesis of this chapter, that is, that generalizations about a disease process can be used as a means of coming to terms with the complexities of that process and its individual manifestations in each patient's world. The ability to do so is, in essence, the foundation of caring for the unique—and total—human being.

A note on the last days of Anne and Sybil provides further understanding of the pathology in question and the individuals involved. Sybil was discharged on a Thursday during the 3-day period of care on which this chapter focuses. Her last morning of care during hospitalization was relatively free of pain and was spent in apparent pleasant anticipation of her return home. She died that weekend of what was believed to be a self-induced, purposeful overdose of the narcotic analgesic methadone. Anne exhibited incredible will to live. Medical consultation revealed that she had made remarkable comebacks in terms of her grave prognosis. The consultation agreed with my opinion that Anne's intense compulsion for organization did not allow her to accept the disorganization of her own body. However, as abdominal involvement increased, Anne made a willful decision that palliative therapy should be discontinued. Her anxiety decreased, and she died while hospitalized. In their unique ways, both Anne and Sybil had come to terms with death.

REFERENCES

1. Brule, G., and others: Drug therapy of cancer, Geneva, 1973, World Health Organization.
2. Capra, L. G.: The care of the cancer patient, London, 1972, Heinemann Medical Books, Ltd.
3. Dickerson, J. W. T.: Nutrition and the cancer patient, The Nursing Mirror and Midwives Journal **135**:39, June 23, 1972.
4. Dickerson, J. W. T.: Nutrition and the cancer patient: food and the aetiology of cancer, The Nursing Mirror and Midwives Journal **136**:33, June 30, 1972.
5. Dickerson, J. W. T.: Nutrition and the cancer patient: metabolic effects of cancer, The Nursing Mirror and Midwives Journal **137**:39, July 7, 1972.
6. French, R. M.: The nurse's guide to

diagnostic procedures, ed. 3, New York, 1971, McGraw-Hill Book Co.

7. Garattini, S., and Franchi, G., editors: Chemotherapy of cancer dissemination and metastases, New York, 1973, Raven Press.
8. Hoch-Ligeti, C.: Laboratory aids in diagnosis of cancer, Springfield, Ill., 1969, Charles C Thomas, Publisher.
9. Kübler-Ross, E.: On death and dying, New York, 1969, The Macmillan Co.
10. Mitchell, P. H.: Concepts basic to nursing, New York, 1973, McGraw-Hill Book Co.
11. Moss, W. T., Brand, W. N., and Battifora, H.: Radiation oncology: rationale, technique, results, ed. 4, Saint Louis, 1973, The C. V. Mosby Co.
12. Oddig, J. A.: American Hospital Formulary Service, vols. 1 and 2, Washington, D.C., 1973, American Society of Hospital Pharmacists.
13. Shafer, K. N., and others: Medical-surgical nursing, ed. 6, Saint Louis, 1975, The C. V. Mosby Co.
14. Weisman, A. D.: On dying and denying: a psychiatric study of terminality, New York, 1972, Behavioral Publications.

ADDITIONAL READINGS

Dao, T. L.: Advances in breast cancer research. In Murphy, G., Pressman, D., and Mirand, E., editors: Perspectives in cancer research and treatment, New York, 1973, Alan R. Liss, Inc.
Graham, R. M.: The cytologic diagnosis of cancer, Philadelphia, 1972, W. B. Saunders Co.
Tarin, D.: Tissue interactions in carcinogenesis, New York, 1972, Academic Press, Inc.
Wissler, R., Dao, T., and Wood, S., editors: Endogenous factors influencing host-tumor balance, Chicago, 1967, The University of Chicago Press.
Wood, S.: Neoplasia and the microcirculation. In Wells, R., editor: The microcirculation in clinical medicine, New York, 1973, Academic Press, Inc.

13 Living with cancer

the rights of the patient and the rights of the nurse

ANN ELISABETH PAULEN

Patient's rights are receiving increasing publicity. Consumers are becoming more vocal in demanding their right to health care that is humane and of high quality. Patients' rights as enumerated by such groups as the American Hospital Association include the following: the right to information about one's condition, the right to give informed consent, the right to confidentiality, and the right to privacy.[1] The observations in this chapter relating to both patients and nurses are an expansion of these rights. They are based on 15 years of experience both with people who are living with cancer and with the nurses who are working with them.

A person learning to live with *any* diagnosis has the right to consideration of psychosocial as well as physical needs, but this is particularly apparent when the patient has cancer. The person who receives the diagnosis of cancer will be experiencing a crisis because of what this diagnosis generally means to the lay public as well as to the medical profession. Cancer is still seen as a killer; the very word connotes pain, prolonged suffering, and death.[2]

What, then, are some of the rights of a person who is coming to terms with the physical and emotional changes that can be brought about by this disease? And how can the nurse ensure the realization of these rights?

One of the foremost rights of the patient is the *right to communication*. This is more than the right to information. It is the right to two-way sharing with the staff. Persons with cancer have often seen changes occur in the communication with those who are close to them. One patient said: "I would like to talk with my husband about how I feel and what I'm thinking when the future looks so uncertain, but he doesn't want to talk about it. He gets upset and silent. My daughter starts to cry every time I bring up the subject, so I really don't feel like I can talk to her either. I have started writing down how I feel in a kind of diary so I can get some of this out of my system." In sharing this experience the patient was able to start communicating with a concerned nurse about how she was feeling in relation to what was happening to her.

Since communication implies involvement of two people, the nurse must take an active role. Listening is vitally important; it is not a passive activity. The patient has a right to a listening ear. The nurse can listen and learn what is on the patient's mind—for example, the patient's perception of the disease and its treatment, as well as fears of sickness, mutilation, financial loss, and/or a change in significant relationships. After one nurse and patient had spent time together discussing the diagnosis of cancer and how the patient could continue therapy at home, the patient said: "You know, there is something that has been on my mind for 3 years. I've wanted to ask, but the nurses always seem so busy, and I suppose the question is silly. A relative died of cancer, and I had to help dispose of his clothes. I gave most of them to the Salvation Army. Do you suppose I caught cancer from my relative and that other people who wore his clothes got cancer because I gave those clothes away?" The nurse took this opportunity to clear up the woman's misconception about the cause of cancer as it relates to communicability. The patient said that she felt comfortable in voicing her long standing concern because the nurse had listened to her, taken her seriously, and discussed questions with her in a matter-of-fact and accepting manner.

The nurse can facilitate communication by being open and honest and caring about the other person. One of the surest ways to cut off communication is to offer blanket reassurance—for example: "Everything is going to be okay; don't worry." When the patient knows that the prognosis is not good or at least is in doubt, such a comment may indicate to the patient that the nurse does not care to enter into an open, meaningful dialogue.

Another way to facilitate communication with patients and let them know that we care about what is happening to them is to validate our observations. We may think that we know what is on a patient's mind because of what we observe. We make our own interpretation of the patient's behavior but fail to validate it with the patient. For example, one day the physicians told a patient that she would be started on combination drug therapy but did not explain further. The nurse observed the patient looking depressed, with her head down, shoulders hunched, and handkerchief clutched in her hand. The nurse thought that it was no wonder the patient was depressed, since she had developed more metastases and had to have her therapy changed, but the nurse decided to validate this assumption and said to the patient: "Mrs. M., you look depressed this morning. What is the trouble?" Mrs. M.: "They told me I have to go on combination therapy." Nurse: "What does that mean to you?" Mrs. M.: "Well, when I was here last year, another patient told me that when they don't know what to do with you, they just mix several drugs together and give it to you. So I guess 'this is it.' " The nurse was able to explain to Mrs. M. that there was a specific reason for each drug in the combination, that other people had responded to this combination, and that there was still hope for control of her cancer even though it could not be cured. The patient's misconception was clarified because the nurse took the initiative to validate an observation of the patient's behavior.

Occasionally, the patient may not respond to the invitation to talk about a problem. For example, a patient may say, "Yes, I am depressed, but I don't want to talk about it." The nurse could answer, "If you would like to talk about it at any time, just let me know." The nurse is respecting the patient's right to privacy and is also communicating a caring attitude toward what the patient is experiencing.

This type of communication often leads to *involvement with staff,* which is another right of patients. Patients have the right to have people on the staff care about what happens to them. They have a right to expect the staff members to share with them as they are sharing personal thoughts and feelings with the staff. For example, a patient who was having a rapid spread of her breast cancer asked a nurse who had returned from having a breast biopsy if she had been scared about the outcome of the biopsy. The nurse said: "Yes, I was scared. I'm not at all sure how I would have reacted if this had turned out to be malignant." This sharing of a personal feeling led to a discussion, tearful at times, of how the patient was struggling to live with her cancer.

Involvement means that a staff member will try to stay with a distressed patient even when it is difficult to do so. It means that the staff member will look the patient in the eye even when the topic is a very emotional one. It means that the staff member will not feel compelled to hide a sympathetic tear, although some will label tears as "unprofessional." Involvement with a patient occurs when the nurse views both of them as human beings. The artificial stereotype of detached, efficient "nurse" and grateful, compliant "patient" fades away.

When we look at the patient as a human being, we can readily acknowledge the patient's *right to participate in decision making* about the care provided. One patient found that he upset the whole ward routine because he wanted to bathe in the evening rather than in the morning as he was "supposed to do." Patients with cancer have said that one of the things that bothers them most is their feeling of lack of control over the progression of the disease process.[3] Thus the patient needs to be able to exert control when possible. Patients can make decisions about the timing of their activities of daily living, about many aspects of their treatment plan, and about how to carry out the medical regimen in a way compatible with their life-style. For example, one 73-year-old widow with metastatic breast cancer was told by the medical staff that she definitely could not live alone. There was a danger of pathologic fracture, and she must be under constant observation. The staff was particularly adamant with this patient because they knew that she had laid new carpet by herself during the week before coming to the hospital. The patient was given no chance to respond to this ultimatum until a nurse sat down to discuss these plans with her. The patient said very matter-of-factly that she would rather die than give up her independence and live with one of her children, even though several of them were willing to have her. She also said, with a twinkle in her eye, "Couldn't I fracture my hip right here in the hospital?" She had a point! She was alert and well oriented, and she was articulate about what her life-style meant to her. The concern about her well-being and the possibilities of what could happen were explained to her. She understood the alternatives and made a choice: she decided to stay alone. The patient and nurse then discussed measures such as adding another phone, delivery of groceries, daily calls from her children, and home evaluation by the local public health nurse to make the home environment as safe as possible for her.

Another right that the patient has is the *right to cope in an individual manner.* An important consideration is the individual patient's perception of cancer. This will be affected by what the patient has read, seen, or experienced. Individual perception will affect the manner of coping. Coping is not inherently "good" or "bad." It is only "different" from one person to another, depending on background, beliefs, etc.

None of us know how we would react if we found ourselves in the patient's situation. We need to give this fact some thought so that we do not confuse our coping mechanisms with the patients', nor place our biases, expectations, and value judgments on the patient. If a person's way of coping appears to be detrimental physically or emotionally, we can discuss it as we see it from our point of view. However, in the last analysis, it is up to the patient to decide and to cope in his own individual way.

Coping mechanisms may vary over time with the same patient and family. For example, a 27-year-old woman recently said that when she had initially received the diagnosis of cancer, it seemed very unreal to her. She was treated with surgery, radiation, and chemotherapy, and she was optimistic about the results of treatment. Then, only 9 months later, she had evidence of recurrence. This time she was angry and questioned why this disease had affected her. She said that it was much harder to accept the recurrence than the original disease. Another patient said, "I thought I had come to terms with this diagnosis, but each time I come into the hospital I have to go through the whole thing again." Thus we may see different reactions while the patient is waiting to be diagnosed, at the time of actual diagnosis, and at the time of recurrence. The intensity of this continuing struggle to learn to live with cancer varies with life events and with the physical and emotional status of the patient over time.

Several patients have said that the most depressing time comes after they return home. In the hospital, personnel are supportive, and they are used to seeing people with radical surgery and the distressing side effects of treatment. However, this feeling of acceptance may change abruptly after discharge. If patients see family life going on about them, and they are not involved in the same way as before, they may become depressed and frustrated. The full realization of change in role, change in significant relationships, and change in self-image may be felt.

The nurse who goes into the home can be very helpful to the patient at this crucial time. The nurse can support both the patient and significant others as they learn to live with the changes in life-style that cancer may have wrought. The patient has a right to this continuity of care between the institution and the community, and the nurse has the responsibility to ensure this right.

The patient has a *right to have his family and significant others considered.*

Sometimes health care workers seem to forget that the patients are in the hospital for only a small segment of their life, and that they are an integral part of a whole social network outside the hospital. People who are important to a patient need to be told more than the perfunctory "his condition is satisfactory." The family members can be given current information about changes in the patient's condition and can be treated as though they are important people to have around. Since most of the attention is on the patient, a family member is often surprised and relieved when a nurse says, "How are *you* getting along?" This simple question gives the family member a chance to have some questions answered and to express feelings about what has been happening in relation to the sick relative. Giving support to the relative in the form of a cup of coffee and a listening ear may in turn enable him to give support to the one who is ill.

Giving and receiving support is a very individual matter. One patient may find family members supportive, whereas another patient may express the desire to be alone during times of stress. The patient and the nurse can work together to assess the situation and plan care.

Now that some of the rights of the patient have been enumerated, let us consider several rights of the nurse, for if the patient has a right to communication and involvement with the staff, the other half of this two-way, sharing relationship must be considered. The nurse is, as is the patient, first and foremost a human being and has the right to be treated as an individual, the right to individual feelings, the right to become involved with people, and the right to receive support from others.

In the context of the patient/nurse relationship, this human being is also a professional member of a health care team and therefore not only has rights but also has responsibilities. The professional nurse has the responsibility to bring not only intelligence and knowledge of nursing intervention but also sensitivity and humanness to patient care. The nurse's feelings in a particular situation are a part of being human. Feelings cannot be controlled, any more than physical characteristics such as the size of one's ears can be controlled. *However,* the nurse can control what *is done with these feelings.* The nurse can think through a situation and consider what would be therapeutic. Thus the professional nurse has the responsibility of combining knowledge of therapeutic intervention with humanness in interacting with others.

There may be many facets to the feelings experienced by a nurse who is working with a person with cancer. As stated before, the nurse has a *right to these feelings.* The feelings are influenced by knowledge about cancer, by experiences in both personal and professional life, and by the attitudes of fellow professionals and the general public. Because many of these feelings may be uncomfortable, the nurse may be reluctant to enter into a sharing, human relationship with a patient.

One frequently expressed feeling is helplessness. When curative therapy is no longer possible and the nurse is called on to be supportive to a person receiving palliative measures only, some nurses feel powerless and ineffective. This feeling of helplessness may be related to the nurse's philosophy of nursing.

Much of the medical profession has "cure" as a goal. In working with people with cancer, we know that although one third of the people are cured, two thirds are not.[4] We will thus be working with many people who are receiving palliative rather than curative therapy. If our goal is "care" rather than "cure," we need not feel helpless and ineffective. We can care for a person until the moment of death. Nurses are familiar with physical comfort measures that let the patient and significant others know we care. Another way to be effective is to promote emotional comfort through the provision of the patient's right to communication, involvement, and individualization of care.

Another uncomfortable feeling expressed by many nurses has been that of frustration or anger with a person who delays in seeking treatment. By coming to us when cure is no longer a possibility, the patient is in a sense making us less effective in our treatment. For example, a woman was admitted with a large, draining chest lesion and grossly edematous arm. Her lesion was diagnosed as advanced cancer of the breast. The staff was aghast that she could wait so long before seeking medical attention. The dismay of the staff was not usually verbally expressed to the patient, but she watched the nurse's facial expression very carefully as her dressings were being changed. In the assessment of this patient's situation, it was discovered that she was the sole support of her family. Her husband was incapacitated by a stroke, and they had no insurance. She felt that she must work as long as she possibly could because the alternative was to go on welfare, and she did not want that. Gaining an appreciation for this women's situation helped to dissipate some of the staff's feelings of anger over her delay. All did not agree with her priorities, but they could work with her more therapeutically rather than having the anger and frustration block communication and involvement.

Another feeling often experienced by the nurse is that of the discomfort of working with a person who is angry. It is normal for the person with cancer to be angry and the question why this should be happening.[5] Even though we know this, it is still uncomfortable to be on the receiving end of the patient's frustration. Again, we need to step back and realize what may be happening so that we can let the patient ventilate feelings. Likewise, the person who is depressed and crying can evoke uncomfortable feelings. We know that this reaction, too, is normal when a person realizes, for example, that his cancer is not curable. However, we often feel the need to "do" something tangible or to "say" something profound. Listening and voicing our concern as previously discussed can be therapeutic for the other person.

Sometimes nurses may feel dishonest and caught in a conspiracy when a decision is made not to tell the patient the diagnosis. This problem seems to be greater when the diagnosis is cancer. The reason lies in the particular aura of fear and anxiety that surrounds this disease entity. Nurses may be able to intervene if the patient is asking questions that indicate that he wants to know or in fact already does know the diagnosis. If those who made the decision have this additional information, they may decide to talk with the patient about the diagnosis of cancer.

Another feeling nurses have experienced and have a right to is that of sadness. When nurses care and have been involved with a patient and significant others, it is certainly normal to be sad if things are not going well for the patient. For example, a terminally ill person with cancer was being transferred to a nursing home. As the nurse was saying goodbye to the patient and his wife, she knew that the patient did not have long to live. All three of them knew it. The nurse said very little. She squeezed the patient's hand and had tears in her eyes as she walked to the waiting ambulance with them. The nurse's feelings of sadness were evidence of her humanness.

We as nurses have the *right to become involved with patients and significant others*. The extent of our involvement will vary from person to person, as it does in our private lives. As with the right to our feelings and the attendant responsibility for what we do with our feelings, the right to become involved carries the responsibility to be therapeutic in our involvement. We can share how we are feeling in a particular situation, but sharing personal experiences may not be particularly beneficial to the patient. For example, a person whom several of the staff had known over a period of a year was trying to decide whether to stop all therapy. At this time her concern was centered on herself. She did not care to discuss anyone or anything else. She had had surgery twice, radiotherapy several times, and three different courses of chemotherapy for her metastatic cancer of the breast. She asked several staff members what they might do in her circumstances. Those who had become involved in a sharing, caring relationship with her expressed their feelings. Some agreed with her desire to stop treatment, and others did not agree. She appreciated their honest sharing on this controversial and emotional matter.

The essence of involvement is *sharing* of one's self as one human being with another human being. Presenting a stereotyped, detached, efficient, one-sided facade to every patient we meet will not result in involvement. Each relationship is a unique one between two people who are different from each other. We not only have the right to become involved; we have the responsibility to become involved. Only then can we give individualized care that is fit for human beings.

As care givers, nurses also have the *right to be treated as individuals*. We are human beings first and then female, male, husband, wife, mother, brother, nurse, etc. We need to acknowledge our individual humanness instead of setting unrealistic and inhuman expectations of ourselves—for example, to have all the answers, to be in control of every situation, to say and do the "right" thing at all times, to like all our patients, or to be completely comprehensive in assessing and meeting every patient's needs. As human beings we all have our strengths and our limitations.

Sometimes we need to withdraw and to renew ourselves in a way that makes sense to us as individuals. For example, a nurse who was working on a cancer ward had 3 patients die in 1 week. As the week progressed, she becaume more and more agitated. It was discovered that she not only was under the emotional strain of experiencing the loss of these patients but was also having problems with a deteriorating marriage. She decided that both personally and professionally she needed to move to an area with less emotional stress until some of her problems could be resolved. A change of assignment was arranged with the help of her supervisor. After she found help for her personal problems, she was again able to reach out to help other people.

The previous example illustrates another right—the *right of the nurse to receive support*. The nurse as well as the patient is part of a larger social network. As much as a nurse tries to leave personal problems at home, it cannot always be done. Supportive people will observe signs of frustration or depression in their co-workers as they will in their patients. It also helps to have the acknowledgement of supervisors that working with people who have cancer can be emotionally hazardous. The nurse who receives support in the form of listening, sharing, and caring is then better able to offer suport to others.

Living with cancer can be facilitated by considering the rights of the patient and the rights of the nurse. Each of us in our own setting can discover innovative ways to put these concepts into practice. We do not need physicians' orders, policy changes, or committee meetings. We do need a willingness to risk involvement and to interact with patients and significant others as fellow human beings. These are, in the last analysis, human rights.

REFERENCES

1. American Hospital Association: a patient's bill of rights, Chicago, 1972.
2. Shepardson, Jan: Team approach to the patient with cancer, American Journal of Nursing **72:**488-491, March, 1972.
3. Abrams, Ruth: The patient with cancer: his changing pattern of communication, New England Journal of Medicine **274:** 317-322, Feb. 10, 1966.
4. American Cancer Society: Cancer facts and figures, New York, 1975.
5. Crary, William, and Gerald Crary: Emotional crises and cancer, CA: A Cancer Journal for Clinicians **24:**36-39, Jan.-Feb., 1974.

14 Pain and the cancer patient

MARYLIN JANE DODD
CAROLYN A. LIVINGSTON

In our clinical experience, the belief that pain is to be expected with cancer has frequently been evident in discussions with colleagues, patients, and families. The actual incidence of pain with cancer is significant; however, it is not present in the frequency professionals and the lay public seem to believe. According to Twycross,[23] 40% of all cancer patients suffer severe pain, and 10% experience pain less intensely. However, the other 50% of all cancer patients have little or no pain or discomfort. Many times the pain is not due to the malignancy itself but to the effects of immobilization, for example.

Interestingly, in reviewing the literature many oncology texts have devoted very little space or none at all to a discussion of cancer patients who experience pain. On one hand, pain is believed to occur with great frequency, and on the other, its frequency and importance are negated.

This chapter will be devoted to those cancer patients who do experience pain and will utilize the nursing process as the organizing approach. Current theories and facts about cancer and pain will be discussed in the section on assessment. The sections on intervention will include discussions of what potentially can be done in the light of our knowledge, including specific clinical examples. Finally, an evaluation of the effectiveness of management of pain in cancer patients will be given.

It is important to establish a baseline knowledge of the relationship between cancer and pain before any systematic, effective assessment can begin. Therefore, the emphasis in the first section of this chapter will be predominantly on theories and facts regarding the cancer patient experiencing *pain*. The deemphasis of cancer knowledge is not intended to negate its importance; it has been discussed in other chapters of this book.

Pain occurs most frequently in cancer of the cervix, lung, rectum, and prostate. It may develop in other types of cancer but is not as common.[22]

Current literature attests to the challenge of caring for the cancer patient, especially in the terminal phase. It also speaks to the difficulty of caring for the patient in severe pain. When these two conditions occur in the same patient, the task is formidable. The whole idea of being in a therapeutic relationship that involves someone who is progressively deteriorating and who has intractable pain strikes directly at the vulnerability of the "I." This could happen to me, and would I have enough courage to see it through?

171

Turnbull[22] states that the terminal phase is the time of crisis. Although the patient fears dying, fear of the *process* of dying, which includes fear of pain, is even stronger. Will I be able to cope with it? Will I be able to obtain sufficient relief? Will my courage fail? Will I lose control? Will others abandon me? This fear of dying can present, and in many instances does present an immensely difficult problem for both patient and nurse.

Much of what we know about pain has evolved from experimental studies. The direct transfer of knowledge resulting from these experimental studies to their application to the clinical situation may be made with certain constraints in mind. Sternbach,[20] Bakan,[1] and, more forcibly, Beecher[3] have voiced opposition to making a total comparison between experimental and clinical pain. In the experimental studies the researcher must abide by humanitarian constraints. The volunteer experimental subjects would not have the same perception of, nor reaction to, the sensation of pain, including its meaning for them and anxiety over its consequences. In the clinical setting the researcher is limited in the experimental controls he can humanly impose. Therefore in reading experimental pain studies, the reader does well to keep these limitations in mind.

PAIN

What is pain? It has been defined as a complex perception; an elementary sensation; an affect (emotion); a noxious stimulus; a neurochemical stress reaction; or a result of internal psychic conflicts, threat, interpersonal manipulation, or the human condition. No one approach is either superior or inferior to another, but each has a part to play in identifying and demonstrating the many components of the concept of pain. In our efforts to understand pain by compartmentalizing, we must be careful not to lose sight of the whole—the person who is experiencing this pain.

Since pain is an abstract term referring to many different real things, such as different personal experiences, different noxious stimuli, and different individual responses, it may be helpful to think of pain as "an abstract concept which refers to (1) a personal, private sensation of hurt, (2) a harmful stimulus which signals current or impending tissue damage, (3) a pattern of responses which operate to protect the organism from harm."[20] Yet, even this abstract concept, when applied to the dying cancer patient, falls short and is incomplete, as will be discussed later.

Chronic pain

Pain provoked by environmental stimuli is to be avoided if at all possible. However, when contact is made between ourselves and the noxious stimuli, a response of withdrawal from that source of pain is automatic. This withdrawal behavior does not effectively work for patients experiencing chronic and protracted pain. Their pain is not perceived as external but as internal, and with these pains there is no object to avoid or withdraw from. The pain becomes part of the core, the essence of the patient. The occupation of the body by this austere, alien force has a tendency, particularly over a period of time, to overwhelm, to totally consume, and to thoroughly exhaust its parent member.

In the light of the devastation occurring within the person experiencing chronic protracted pain, it is small wonder that in time his interaction with his environment alters. He loses interest in his surroundings, and the pain becomes the consumer of his energies and attention. The pain can completely dominate his life to the exclusion of everything else.

"At first the pain is dull—in many instances it progresses to severe, relentless, agonizing, intractable suffering that eventually causes physical and mental depletion. Finally, these poor sufferers lose all interest. Pain becomes a consuming problem which dominates their lives."[9]

As if the exposure to this horrendous experience were not enough, there is a perpetration of the increasing pain by a cyclic bioneurologic feedback mechanism. According to Bonica,[8] this feedback mechanism is initiated or maintained in a cycle by persistent reflex responses to trauma or disease that are associated with sympathetic hyperactivity, vasoconstriction, local ischemia, and accumulation of metabolites of painful stimulation.

There is the belief that elderly patients have an increased tolerance to pain. Since life is filled with pain in one form or the other, exposure over time leads to the development of coping behaviors. To the majority of the elderly, pain is no stranger. Contrary to popular belief, however, Bonica[8] believes that patients do not become more accustomed to chronic pain but instead become even more sensitive and suffer more. Physical and mental depletion produced by protracted pain, whether moderate or severe, varies widely from person to person. Nevertheless, these depletions are present to some degree in all.

How untimely it is that a cancer patient has to deal with profound suffering and depletion of body energies at a time when some incredibly difficult work awaits, that is, progressing through the termination of his own life. Bakan[1] most precisely summed it up when he said, "Pain and mortality make up the tragedy of man."

Loneliness of pain

Pain is a highly subjective, private, and personal experience. As helping professionals, regardless of the amount of empathy we have or our personal past experiences with pain, we cannot experience another's pain. Pain can only be communicated imperfectly, and the more profound the pain, the more it defies communication through words or actions.[20] "One is never so incredibly alone as when he is in pain." The often futile attempts to make others understand and the patient's diminished interactions with the environment reinforce this loneliness.

Search for meaning in pain

The search to the question "Why me?" is twofold for the patient who has both terminal cancer and protracted pain. The termination of life is one of the most sobering experiences all of us will eventually face. Yet, above and beyond this human plight, to live out one's remaining time in intense and intractable pain demands interpretation. Involvement in a therapeutic relationship with someone in search of the answer to the question "why" has the tendency to stir up incredible feelings of helplessness in health professionals. We do not have the answer, or even if we do possess our own answer to this question, it cannot be given to another as a solution to his quest. In a conversation with a student, one of us (M.J.D.) asked how a nurse could help the dying patient search and find a satisfactory answer. After much thought the student later came back and said: "It is up to the individual who is actually dying and in pain to answer the question of 'why.' It is, strictly speaking, between him, his pain, his dying, and God. We as caring professionals can be with him and support him in the best way we know how, but the vast bulk of the work is his and his alone. We can only indirectly participate at best."

The search for the answer to the question of "why" is made more difficult when we look at the physiologic protective function of the nature of pain. One of the major functions of pain is to cause the organism to withdraw from sources of damage, but with the cancer patient the withdrawal response does not apply because of the internal nature of the pain, as mentioned earlier. Pain is a warning signal against damage to the body tissues and cells. In the terminal cancer patient we are already aware of the destruction taking place. What is the point of this pain, the presence of which impairs the patient's ability to focus on little else, to think clearly, to resolve the termination of life, and to say good-byes.

In Sternbach's presentation, the mechanics of the search for the "why" include regression, punishment, guilt, loneliness, and abandonment. "When we are feeling extended pain, before we have yet reached exhaustion, our thoughts and actions take on a decidedly childish turn."[20] As a child we search for what we have done to deserve such pain. Then comes contriteness and as contriteness fails, the child searches for the reason the parent is punishing us so, and later pleads to the parent for mercy. The fantasy of punishment in association with pain has two important components:

1. The threat of bodily harm by the punitive parent
2. Aloneness and abandonment by that parent[20]

Other areas explored in the timeless search for the "why" include Christianity and existentialism. Bakan[1] believes that one could very well argue that one of the major psychologic uses of Christianity has been to overcome the essential loneliness and privacy of pain. The existentialists bring other aspects of the understanding of pain into focus. Their thesis is that pain is the essence of the human condition, and that when we are experiencing this pain we are supremely alone; yet through this experience we are united to the rest of suffering humanity. Buytendijk[10] infers from the effects of pain experiences that it is a potentially character-enabling phenomenon, and thus the search for the meaning of pain continues.

Individuality of pain response

Individual emotional or physical responses to distress do not have a direct or equal relationship to the intensity of the pain sensation. There are many factors that play a part in the individual's reactions to pain, including the individual's unique personality, perception, emotional state, past experiences, and ethnic background.

Before discussing these factors, it would be useful to review the difference between pain threshold and pain tolerance. "Pain threshold refers to the intensity at which a person first makes a pain response, when it first catches his attention and the message of pain is consciously noted. Pain tolerance is the duration of time or the intensity at which a subject accepts a stimulus above the pain threshold before making a verbal or overt escape response."[20]

Personality characteristics influence how individuals perceive, interpret, and respond to the sensory stimulation of pain. This individuality has been demonstrated in many experimental studies. Witkin and colleagues,[24] in their development of field dependence–field independence theory, have found that, in making perceptual judgments, people vary in the extent to which they depend on environmental stimuli. In their study, subjects are asked to align a rod to a gravitational vertical line in a darkened room with no other cues except a tilted frame surrounding the rod. Subjects who succeed in aligning the rod vertically are field independent (they use internal cues, ignoring the tilted frame). Subjects who align the rod in accordance with the frame are called field dependent (they are influenced by the tilted frame). Field-dependent persons are more aggressive, have a larger repertoire of coping behaviors, and show more differentiation in their responses. Field-dependent persons are more passive and accepting, and show less differentiation in their responses. In regard to pain, field-dependent subjects appear to be less responsive to pain and at the same time are more influenced by external stimuli. Manipulation of the environment for these field-dependent individuals could be useful in the management of their clinical pain if the results of experimental studies hold up in the clinical situation.[5]

People vary in the accuracy with which they perceive the intensity of sensory stimulation. Researchers, notably Petrie,[19] have demonstrated a relationship between response to pain and personal estimate of size and intensity of sensory data. Three categories of subjects has come out of Petrie's experiments:

> Reducer—tends to subjectively decrease the sensory data that is perceived
> Augmenter—tends to subjectively increase the sensory data that is perceived
> Moderator—tends to neither increase nor decrease the sensory data that is perceived

Consequently, the reducer has the greater tolerance to pain, due to the tendency to decrease the perception of the stimulation. This tendency to diminish sensory data can work against the reducer in the situations of isolation and confinement, which occur in chronic illness, hospitalization, and the process of dying.

Another area of research focusing on the way different people interact with their environment has combined the use of the extroversion-introversion scale with the concept of neuroticism.[11] Extroversion refers to the outgoing, uninhibited, impulsive, and sociable inclinations of a person, and introversion is the other end of the extroversion scale. Neuroticism refers to the general emotional overresponsiveness and liability to neurotic breakdown under stress.

Lynn and Eysenck[15] obtained a very significant positive correlation in their research of extroversion and pain tolerance. The most extroverted subjects tolerated pain for the longest period, and there was significant negative correlation of neuroticism with pain tolerance.

In experimental study, Bond[6] found communication about pain to be related to extroversion-introversion. Subjects who are more introverted are less likely to report pain, even though the intensity of the pain experience is greater than that experienced by the extroverts.

In the light of these facts, the implications for nursing are clear. Reliance on the patient's verbal reporting of pain cannot totally be depended on to determine when pain relief is warranted. Introverted patients may even deny the existence of pain when asked. With these patients, other pain assessment criteria must be used. Another explanation of why, when several persons are exposed to the same painful stimuli, they will respond differently, lies in the structural differences of their nervous systems. In addition, human beings are the sum total of all their experiences, and if those life experiences have included pain, present or future confrontations with pain will be affected by the past. The presence of malnutrition, anemia, fatigue, or emotional turmoil tends to decrease the individual's tolerance of pain. Ethnic factors influence the acceptability of expressing pain—not pain tolerance. Some ethnic groups allow more freedom of expression, whereas others maintain and reinforce stringent rules for nonexpression, either verbally or behaviorally.

The positive relationship between anxiety and pain has been reported in many research studies. Anxiety intensifies the pain experience and response. Caring for a patient having intense pain is challenging enough without having to cope with a large dose of highly contagious anxiety. This combination of conditions occurring in the same patient has the tendency to bring out the "flight" mechanism in most health professionals.

Meaning of pain

In an earlier discussion the patient's search for the answer to the question "why" was presented. This discussion is a continuation of that theme, for whether or not the patient has established a satisfactory response to the question of "why," the fact remains that pain does have some meaning for him. The progressive, protracted pain of the patient with metastatic cancer symbolizes a process that will end in death. The ever-present pain is a constant reminder of the dying process, and the successful use of denial in the terminal cancer patient does not appear to work nearly as well in the presence of excruciating pain. The heavy toll on body energies taken by pain leaves little strength for mobilizing or sustaining defense mechanisms.

ASSESSMENT

With the establishment of a baseline knowledge of the relationship between cancer and pain, it will be useful now to specifically focus on clinical assessment. In the process of gathering data at the bedside, it is helpful to keep in mind some specific questions to ask the patient in order to construct an accurate personal history of the pain. Particularly pertinent is the determination of the location, duration, quality, intensity, and type of pain experienced. What aggravates or relieves it? Systematizing these data facilitates the devising of an individualized plan for relief.

Petrie, in her research, has devised the following assessment tool for registering the response to pain*:

	None	Slight	Moderate	Severe	Agony
1. Involuntary verbal expressions of pain					
2. Demand for analgesics					
3. Spontaneous reports of pain					
4. Restlessness					
5. Squirming, stiffening, gripping					
6. Interference with breathing					
7. Interference with talking					
8. Physical signs of pain (e.g., blanching, sweating, tremors, dilation of pupils)					
9. Interference with sleeping					
10. Interference with eating and other daytime activities					

*From Petrie, A.: Individuality in pain and suffering, Chicago, 1967, The University of Chicago Press.

NURSING INTERVENTION

The nurse can help the patient cope with the meaning of pain and death. Providing psychologic support includes "being" with the patient, listening very carefully, and trying to understand his individual perception of what is happening. McCaffery[16] presents the patient's needs for respect, encouragement, and high but realistic expectations. Benoliel and Crowley[5] present another element that is relevant to the psychologic needs of a patient with pain—the concept of "staying." "Staying is not so much the actual physical presence—though at times this is part of it—but 'staying' in the sense of being open or available to the patient. For the nurse to stay confident that one is helping, that what one does is meaningful to oneself as well as to the patient, that one is genuine, and real, and present when needed is essential." The consequence of inadequately providing psychologic support is an aggravation of the pain because the "hope, understanding, and personal interest have been withheld."[14] The goal of pain management is to "conserve the patient's physical, mental, moral resources and his social usefulness as long as possible."[18]

To provide for the patient's physiologic needs, it is essential to account for a variety of different factors, which would include the following:

1. Teaching a patient about the pain being experienced
2. Providing for adequate analgesia
3. Providing for a variety of sensory inputs
4. Facilitating the patient's rest, relaxation, and sleeping patterns
5. Encouraging adequate nutrition, hydration, and elimination
6. Providing good personal hygiene for the patient and cleanliness of the surroundings

Patient teaching

Not knowing about pain tends to increase the degree of anxiety, which, in turn, magnifies the intensity of the pain response. Therefore, giving the patient the physiologic reasons for the experience of pain will diminish anxiety. Adequate preparation prior to painful treatments and/or procedures has the same effect. The nurse should assess the patient's pattern of handling pain and the factors that influence the patient's responses to the pain experience. This assessment will effect what, how, and when the nurse teaches the patient about pain.[16]

Analgesia

In the area of providing for adequate analgesia, we in the nursing profession have many "hang ups." The attitude toward the patient who is experiencing pain determines how the nurse copes with the patient's need for pain relief.

Morgan has aptly pointed out two different attitudes in providing analgesia. The first is the "raw guts" approach—suffering is seen as good, and as something to be respected, and the unstated "bravery" involved is strongly reinforced. In the "peace at any price" approach, it is believed either that the patient does not have the courage to cope with the pain or that we in the therapeutic relationship do not have the time nor the inclination to find alternative mechanisms for pain relief.[17]

In reviewing the literature, one can see that what is most important in the effective management of pain is that the patient receives adequate relief—that he is neither "snowed" with the potency of the dosage nor denied any relief at all. It is difficult to determine the optimum dosage for each patient. As the patient's physical and mental condition deteriorates and the pain becomes more protracted and severe, potent and frequently given analgesics are more commonly used. In our clinical experience the fear that the cancer patient may become an addict has frequently been voiced. This preoccupation with not making the patient an addict did in many instances become an obsession. The question is: Why is this of concern? Is it not our goal to provide for the patient's adequate analgesia, especially in the terminal phase? Lamberton[13] has found that "drug addiction very seldom is a problem, and apart from savage pains, most can be controlled with less than 15 mg of morphine/diacetylmorphine every four hours, the dose creeping up to perhaps double that as the pain worsens shortly before death."

Numerous personal documentations in the literature speak to the agony of the patient's having to wait for the nurse to actually administer the analgesia after his initial request. This waiting is intolerable. When the patient is experiencing immense pain, the accuracy of time perception is greatly reduced. A wait of only 10 minutes can seem endless.

One of the most notable institutions in the management of pain of cancer patients is St. Christopher's Hospice, in Sydenham, England, founded by Cecily Saunders. She uses two concepts: (1) the human-to-human approach, which is central, and (2) involving the patient in determining the potency and frequency of the analgesic. This opportunity to participate in pain management gives the patient security in the fact that adequate relief will be given when it is needed. The analgesic is routinely given at prescribed times at the patient's request, negating the "waiting" phenomenon.

Twycross[23] states that morphine, even when correctly used, is not a panacea for terminal pain. There is a small group of 1% who receive only slight relief from morphine, and 20% more who fail to receive complete relief.

Other examples of the hospice approach to care of the terminally ill include St. Joseph's in the Hackney section of London; Hospice in New Haven, Connecticut; St. Luke's Hospital in New York; and committed planning in San Francisco and Seattle. It is a sad commentary that there are at this time so few institutions that provide such individualized care for cancer patients, particularly in the area of pain control.

Sensory inputs

Providing a variety of sensory inputs may make the pain more bearable and has particular importance for patients who can be described as perception reducers.[19] The isolation and confinement frequently experienced in hospitals during the process of dying limit the amount of varied sensory data that are available to be perceived.

Previously we have mentioned the importance of "staying" and "being," but they may not be enough to comfort a dying and pain-wracked patient. The judicial use of touch can augment our mere presence and is especially important in the terminal phase, when the patient's tendency to withdraw and to be lost within himself is most acute. The use of tactile stimulation as a source of sensory input can be used during the duration of the dying process. Comfort measures such as a backrub, a cool cloth on the patient's forehead, and moist heat for contracted muscles all have a physiologic and psychologic benefit. Knowing the patient's individual preference for other forms of sensory data is useful in deciding what to provide in the way of diversional activity.

Rest and sleep

The tremendous cost of severe pain to the patient's energies has already been discussed. The incredible work the cancer patient must do in the termination of life has been well documented in the literature. The presence of extreme fatigue would seem to be the plight of the dying patient with cancer, and this exhaustion leaves the patient less able to cope with pain.

Therefore, providing the opportunity for rest, relaxation, and sleep is necessary. Several mechanisms, together with the use of analgesia, are important. For example, rhythmic breathing similar to that being used in natural childbirth may help the patient to relax. The use of yoga exercises and transcendental meditation may also be helpful, especially if the patient has mastered these techniques prior to his health crisis. Involve the patient in deciding how to pace the care given. The institutions must allow for individual preferences and not be caught up in having the patient eating breakfast, taking medication, bathing, and making the bed all before 10 o'clock in the morning so that he can be at radiation therapy by 10:15 A.M.

Possible suggestions for providing a patient with restful sleep include minimizing institutional noise, repositioning as needed, and providing effective sedation in combination with an adequate analgesic state, repeating as necessary throughout the night. Verify with the patient whether sleep has been restful. Do not rely on doorway observations to determine that the patient "slept well." Alternatives to a sedative—for example, alcohol, warm milk, or tea—can be determined by patient preference.

Nutrition

Because the cancer patient's condition is disabling and deteriorating, more than adequate nutritional and fluid intake is paramount. This presents an immense challenge to the nurse, since many of these patients, because of the disease or the therapy, are anorexic. Abiding by patient preferences enhances the probability of adequate nutrition. Having consultations with the dietitian assures patient preference and enriched nutritional intake. Eating is work for these patients. Allowing an hour for rest prior to each meal may conserve the energy needed to accomplish the work of eating.

It goes without saying that fluid depletion and constipation can be sources of pain for the immobilized cancer patient.

Personal hygiene

Personal hygiene is of great importance when the deteriorating state of the body is considered. The patient's debilitated state decreases his resistance to environmental organisms. As the patient loses energy and becomes less mobile, the nurse must plan to prevent respiratory complications, skin breakdown, and urinary tract infection. In addition, certain neoplasms produce a typical cancer smell that is distressing to the patient, the family, and the hospital staff. Measures to diminish this odor include locating the source and correcting the situation if possible. Camouflaging the odor with the use of heavy scents and perfumes is to be avoided. If the odor is impossible to remove, ensure adequate ventilation of the room, frequent bathing, and use of a naturally scented deodorizer.

MEDICAL INTERVENTION

Medical intervention of pain in cancer patients has two foci: (1) to cure or decrease the neoplasm and (2) to treat symptomatically. Measures to accomplish the first include radiation, hormonal therapy, chemotherapeutic drugs, and/or palliative surgery. The symptomatic relief provided by the medical profession includes the use of analgesics, regional nerve blocks, and/or neurosurgery.[7,9,18]

REFERENCES

1. Bakan, D.: Disease pain and sacrifice, Chicago, 1968, The University of Chicago Press.
2. Beecher, H. K.: Generalization from pain of various types and diverse origins, Science **130**:267, 1959.
3. Beecher, H: K.: Measurement of subjective responses: quantitative effect of drugs, New York, 1959, Oxford University Press.
4. Beecher, H. K.: Increased stress and effectiveness of placebos and active drugs, Science **132**:91, 1960.
5. Benoliel, J. Q., and Crowley, D. M.: The patient in pain: new concepts. In Proceedings of the National Conference on Cancer Nursing, New York, 1974, American Cancer Society, Inc.
6. Bond, M. R.: The relation of pain of the Eysenck Personality Inventory, Cornell Medical Index and Whiteley Index of Hypochondrosis, The British Journal of Psychiatry **119**:675, Dec., 1971.
7. Bonica, J. J.: Pain associated with cancer and other neoplastic diseases. In The management of pain, Philadelphia, 1953, Lea & Febiger.
8. Bonica, J. J.: Fundamental considerations of chronic pain therapy. Postgraduate Medicine **53**:81, May, 1973.
9. Bonica, J. J., and Backup, P. H.: Control of cancer pain, Northwest Medicine **54**:22, Jan., 1955.
10. Buytendijk, F. J. J.: Pain: Its modes and functions, translated by E. Osheel, Chicago, 1962, The University of Chicago Press.
11. Eysenck, H. J., and Eysenck, S. B. G.: Manual Eysenck personality inventory, San Diego, Calif., 1968, Educational and Industrial Testing Service.
12. Gray, R. V.: Dealing with dying, Nursing '73 **3**:26, June, 1973.
13. Lamberton, R.: Care of the dying, Nursing Times **69**:56, Jan. 11, 1973.
14. Lemon, H. M.: Control of pain in metastatic cancer, Journal of Chronic Diseases **4**:84, July, 1956.
15. Lynn, R., and Eysenck, H. J.: Tolerance for pain, extroversion and neuroticism, Perception Motor Skills **12**:161, 1961.
16. McCaffery, M.: Nursing management of the patient with pain, Philadelphia, 1972, J. B. Lippincott Co.
17. Morgan, A.: Minor tranquilizers, hypnotics and sedatives, American Journal of Nursing **73**:1220, July, 1973.
18. Murphy, T. M.: Cancer pain, Postgraduate Medicine **53**:187, May, 1973.
19. Petrie, A.: Individuality in pain and suffering, Chicago, 1967, The University of Chicago Press.
20. Sternbach, R. A.: Pain: a psychophysiological analysis, New York, 1968, Academic Press, Inc.
21. Sternbach, R. A.: Strategies and tactics in the treatment of patients with pain. In Crue, B. L., editor: Pain and suffering, selected aspects, Springfield, Ill., 1970, Charles C Thomas, Publisher.
22. Turnbull, F.: Pain and suffering in cancer, Canadian Nurse **67**:28, Aug., 1971.
23. Twycross, R. G.: Principles and practices of the relief of pain in terminal cancer, Update, July, 1972.
24. Witkin, H. A., and others: Personality through perception, New York, 1954, Harper & Row, Publishers.
25. Witkin, H. A., and others: Psychological differentiation, New York, 1962, John Wiley & Sons, Inc.

15 Communicating care

PEGGY JUNE NASLUND NELSON

> Unforeseen and unprepared for, the disease had come upon him, a
> happy man with few cares, like a gale in the space of two weeks.
>
> Alexander Solzhenitsyn
> *Cancer Ward*

What comes to your mind when you hear the word *cancer?* Fear? Suffering?
Death? I remember perfectly the feelings I experienced many months ago, when
the image of myself as a healthy, 23-year-old nurse became a distorted picture of
an amputee with cancer. In 2 days I progressed from a cold, to a chest x-ray
examination, to the discovery of a tumor in my left shoulder. I was reassured that
the tumor was benign and that it could be excised locally. Two days after what I
thought was a local excision, my physician explained to me that I had a chondro-
sarcoma. Four days later my arm, scapula, and clavicle were removed. My life was
at a crisis point. Now, 18 months later, I am writing this chapter to identify the
stages of such a crisis. It is written as a guideline for nurses—facilitators for movement through crisis. These guidelines come from the needs I experienced as a patient, and the emotions I have identified as a nurse working with the cancer victim.

Crisis is defined by Webster as "the decisive moment or an emotionally
significant event or radical change in a person's life." It was the culmination of
every emotion I had ever experienced. It is displayed differently in every patient.
Many times the crisis is difficult to identify, but the nurse should look for the
signs of a crisis in every newly diagnosed cancer patient. This is an opportune
time for crisis intervention. A crisis is described by Ruben[3] as "an organism's
inability to maintain behavioral equilibrium." Intervention is the attempt to help
patients and families adjust to the present situation and return to their previous
state of equilibrium. It includes identifying the problem and formulating a plan
for solving that problem.

Kübler-Ross in *On Death and Dying,*[1] gives a thorough explanation of the
stages experienced by the dying patient as the situation is realized and accepted,
and discusses common communication techniques used in each stage. These steps
compare closely to the grieving process of the cancer patient. They are hysteria,
denial, anger, bargaining, depression, and acceptance. In a recent video tape recording called *How Could I Not Be Among You?* a young poet, Ted Rosenthal,
discussed his feelings after being diagnosed as having acute leukemia. He said
that the nurses told him he would go through this stage and that state—"every-

body does." Later he said, "They were right." He did pass through a series of stages, predictable in their happening but not in their symptomatology. Because we are all individuals, the stages become peculiar to each of us as individuals.

HYSTERIA

Hysteria is the first emotion I experienced when I was told that I had cancer. This stage is easily identified by the nurse. Some patients cry and scream. In drastic contrast, others become mute and unresponsive.

Miss D., a 14-year-old with osteosarcoma, illustrates the latter response. Immediately after being told that her leg would be removed because of a tumor, Miss D. sat unresponsive and staring. When I entered her room, I did not know what to say.

Both types of hysterical response are difficult to handle. The initial interaction is the hardest. Patients need a hand to hold even if it is a stranger's hand—it is a source of comfort and strength. Just sitting close to the patient can convey a willingness to share in the patient's pain.

The physician should not expect the patient or the family to understand or remember all the facts and details during this stage. There is a period of adjustment to just the word *cancer* and the fear it evokes. The nurse should be a resource for all these facts because the patient will later ask many questions.

Remain calm. Sit down so that your knees do not shake. Cry if you feel like crying, but do not run away from the patient. The nurse determines the approach that the other members of the health team will use. The nurse assistant, the chaplain, and the social worker all receive their cues from the nurse.

At this point I would like to interject that these stages are listed in the order through which I passed when I found I had cancer. Not every patient goes through the stages in this order, nor does every patient go through all the stages. Every patient is an individual and adjusts as such. The stages are listed with the symptoms that are most commonly seen. In trying to explain my own reaction to cancer in this chapter, I have cited several other examples of patients whose experiences also help to illustrate some of the various aspects of each stage that I experienced. I introduce these examples to point out how the nurse can best help the individual at each stage.

DENIAL

The second stage is denial. I denied the situation, shouting: "No, this isn't true. It can't be me." In addition to such obvious forms of denial, nurses may find patients making unrealistic plans. Some patients covertly deny reality by never mentioning the words *cancer* or *surgery*. Their conversation involves other people, never themselves.

I met Mr. K. 2 weeks after he had had an above-the-knee amputation for osteosarcoma. The nurses were concerned that he was not beginning to accept the loss of his leg. During my first visit, Mr. K. was cheerful. In a matter of minutes he was explaining to me how he was going to become a track star. I am not sure how strongly he believed this, but he continued to make his plans. Mr. K. talked about pole vaulting. He occasionally asked me for confirmation of his ability to pole-vault but never gave me the opportunity to answer his question. About certain subjects, such as swimming, he did not ask me whether or not he would be able to perform. He simply stated such performance as a positive fact.

In addition to his positive attitude, Mr. K. never spoke of being fitted for a prosthesis. He never complained of pain, and his mood was elated, as though nothing had happened. It is as though patients in denial are saying, "The tests were wrong; the doctor is lying to me."

Another patient in this stage was a young woman who had undergone a recent mastectomy. She never spoke of her surgery or future treatment, and she changed the topic of conversation whenever it became personal or threatening.

The approach to use is honesty. Never agree with a patient's fantasy plans. It is particularly important to be honest when patients ask for reassurance concerning the future.

Confronting the patient with reality is another way of dealing with denial. This approach is essential for the patient who continues for days and sometimes weeks without acknowledging the fact that he has cancer. An approach we have found to be useful is saying to the patient, "I know everything is very difficult for you, but you do have cancer, and there are arrangements and decisions to make."

Patients are not alone in their use of denial. Nurses use denial as a defense mechanism to protect themselves, and they allow patients to continue denying because it is not easy for a patient to deal with cancer. I am amazed that a 22-year-old woman can go to surgery for the removal of a massive uterine tumor without a single word charted about her psychologic state. I have heard staff nurses say: "Well, she is accepting it beautifully. She's so cheerful." I question how well she is accepting it. I wonder how many staff members giving her physical care even mentioned her disease, her prognosis, or her husband's feelings. With this patient an approach could be as simple as saying, "Aren't you afraid?"

The manner in which one confronts a patient is important. Never use a loud, angry, or hostile tone of voice. The patient should be confronted by someone who has worked with him and whom he trusts. The confrontation may take the form of a question, such as: "It is difficult for me to understand how you can be cheerful after losing your leg. Could you help me understand how you feel?" Of course, there is no pat phrase, since every situation is different. In many texts on care of the cancer patient, confrontation is minimized and even refuted as useless. Actually, there is no evidence to prove whether or not confrontation helps a patient move through the denial stage. There is also no proof that a patient should not stay in this stage; however, the patient should have the truth and the opportunity to choose acceptance or denial.

ANGER

The third stage of a crisis is anger. The physician, the nurse, and the family are commonly the targets. I became angry at some nonexistent figure because I felt the need to blame someone who would not strike back at me. Patients say hateful things, become demanding, and seem totally unreasonable about the simplest matters. There is often a drastic mood change.

After a kidney biopsy Mr. E. became demanding and arrogant. His complaints included every nurse who cared for him, as well as members of his family. He expected to have a refrigerator in his room, and he did not like his roommate. With much embarrassment his wife apologized for him and tried to explain that "this isn't like him at all." Unfortunately, the staff failed to recognize that his reaction was caused by fear. Mr. E. angered them all.

When the anger of a patient is directed toward the nurse, there is nothing to do but refuse to retaliate. She must prove to the patient that she will accept his expressions of anger without making judgments.

BARGAINING

The next stage is bargaining. I remember thinking that I would give up my arm if only I could live. Certainly the bargain was not reasonable, since I was going to lose my arm either way, but somehow it made dealing with the amputation easier. It also served to postpone dealing with the cancer. Patients often ask for promises, such as: "Can you promise me that there will be no pain?" or "Promise me that I won't die." Some patients try to bargain with the doctors or nurses. Others call out to the previously mentioned nonexistent figure as though that person could take away all that had happened.

The nurse's role may be minute at this point, unless the patient tries to bargain for promises of health. It is difficult for the nurse to be honest when the prognosis is poor, since the nurse often feels a need to heal all. It is essential to avoid false promises. I often respond by saying, "I want to help in any way I can, but I cannot promise you that there will be no pain."

DEPRESSION

When the patient realizes that denying and bargaining do not make the cancer go away, he often retreats into depression. The nurse will observe a drastic change in mood, a decrease in appetite and activity, a lack of eye contact, and frequent requests for medication. Depressed patients have little to say to the nurse. In fact, unless prodded, they will usually say nothing.

For many cancer patients depression is the biggest problem. It also creates the greatest problem for the family because they cannot understand the patient's behavior. For example, a man may continually cry, or a woman may talk about never taking care of her children again. Most patients think that a diagnosis of cancer automatically means that they will die. To many it also means endless suffering.

Many patients react immediately, whereas others become depressed long after being diagnosed. I went for approximately 8 months without depression, possibly because of my immediate return to work. I did not allow myself any time to become depressed. After 8 months I began to think about everything that had happened and everything I could no longer do. I then felt sorry for myself. I could not understand why I felt so terrible, and I experienced a lack of energy and interest. I kept thinking that I had the flu. Every morning at 4 o'clock I would awaken, crying, because I did not want to go to work.

Mr. B., a patient with adenocarcinoma, tried desperately to cover his depression. Whenever a nurse was in the room he was joking and laughing. At one point I asked whether there was anything he feared. He promptly told me that he had no fears. Then he began to cry, and said, "I just want to live." He gave me two responses: the first, the one he thought he should give, was that he was not afraid; the second, the one that expressed his feelings, was that he feared death.

The approach to use with depression is patience. The nurse may be instrumental in helping the patient and the family understand that it is normal to feel some depression and that it is normal to cry. The patient should be encouraged to talk about his feelings. Time should be spent with him, and the nurse should sit beside him on the bed, or should pull a chair close so that the patient and the nurse are physically on the same level. The nurse should communicate to the patient a desire to understand and to help. Making sure that the patient knows the nurse's name, first and last, helps to establish rapport. The patient should know how to get in touch with the nurse if support is needed.

An appreciable amount of time can be spent with the patient and the family each day. Many nurses use the excuse of lack of time, but good use can be made of only 5 or 10 minutes. The nurse should not take anything into the room, since equipment in the hands of a nurse gives too many excuses for leaving. It gives the impression that there are many other things to do. How many times has the nurse heard a patient say, "Oh, I don't want to bother you because I know you are busy"? Let the patient know you want to make time for him because he is important.

The nurse must remain honest and human. Shed a tear, or touch a hand. It is permissible to say, "I don't know what to say." Patients do not expect nurses to be perfect, but they do expect them to be honest. I would like to note here that depression once worked through may recur. It can become evident for no apparent reason or when the patient needs a reaffirmation of the diagnosis and the prognosis.

One way to alleviate the anxiety that produces depression is to give the patient an active part to play in the follow-up treatment. With patients on chemotherapy, common symptoms and side effects should be explained, and the patient can be instructed as to what can be done about them. Patients should be allowed to look at their x-ray films and should be given an explanation of what the films mean.

This technique of giving patients information about themselves has been helpful in alleviating fear.

ACCEPTANCE

The cancer patient can reach a stage of acceptance in which he becomes most like his former self. I reached acceptance when, after surgery, I realized that I was the same person as before, that I still had my job, and that those around me still cared for me.

Another specific sign of acceptance is the point at which the patient can talk freely about the disease without any false hopes. At this stage the patient starts asking questions about what is going to happen and what the treatment will involve. Until the patient reaches the acceptance stage, the nurse may be uneasy, not knowing what to say or how to act.

The family, too, must achieve acceptance. The family's acceptance may be fostered by the nurse, particularly if the family members are given a part in the care of the patient. They will be helpful in recognizing the stages through which the patient is proceeding and the patient's return to his normal self. Soliciting their help in this way can open up the communication lines between the nurse and the family.

HOPE

The last stage of adjustment is hope. As stated earlier, many patients think that cancer always means death. In some cases this is true, but for many patients the prognosis is excellent. Hope for those with a good prognosis might include returning to job and family. For myself, hope was contained in a new zeal for living and a future containing reasonable goals. I have seen this same type of reaction in patients who realize that they are indeed vulnerable but are determined to make full the life they have.

There is also a stage of hope for the dying patient—hope for a peaceful death. The acceptance and hope of the dying patient are displayed by the patient's active support of the nurse and family throughout the dying process. It is ironic that the patient is the supporter, but it must be realized that the patient is the one who has worked through all the stages.

SUMMARY

A nurse cannot force a patient into the stages discussed by Kübler-Ross. Much of the movement takes place inexplicably inside the patient. What the nurse can do is act as a facilitator, creating an open environment and accepting the feelings of the patient and family.

I have listed some of the techniques that can be useful in work with cancer patients. These techniques may vary from nurse to nurse and from patient to patient. The correctness of the nurse's response lies not only in what is said but how it is said. Spontaneity and honesty should be the aim of communication. The utilization of these techniques creates an environment conducive to reaching acceptance.

The nurse also needs an outlet for frustrations and fears. If a patient's situation is upsetting, it should be discussed with someone who is not involved with the patient. Someone else may be able to suggest new approaches for care and understanding; nurses should not expect to have all the answers.

A group discussion about the patient, early in the hospitalization, is a means of alleviating some of the fear. The conference would include all health personnel associated with the patient. At this time the patient's diagnosis, prognosis, and course of treatment should be discussed. Such a discussion will not only give the nurse a better understanding, but it will also help in answering any questions the patient might have.

Another topic for group discussion is the patient's and family's understanding of the illness, and the plans to explain the same. The nurse should have fewer fears after this discussion. It would alleviate the anxiety created by not knowing what the patient and family knows, by not understanding a diagnosis or prognosis, and by giving the nurse time to talk.

A separate conference could include the nurse, physician, patient, and family. In addition to the diagnosis, prognosis, and treatment, the nurse could explain to the patient what the daily care would include. At the same time the patient could give the staff an idea of what his needs and expectations are. All of this information could certainly help in formulating a plan of total care.

The key factor in intervening in a crisis is open communication between the nurse and the patient. A physician recently laughed at my seriousness about the necessity for interpersonal communication, saying that communication was nothing more than shouting at a person at the end of the hall and having the person shout back. The physician may be right. The important thing is that someone listen and respond to that shouting person at the other end of the hall. He may be shouting for help, and nurses can help by using communication to respond to the cancer patient's needs.

REFERENCES

1. Kübler-Ross, E.: On death and dying, New York, 1969, The Macmillan Co.
2. Peck, A.: Emotional reactions to having cancer, CA: A Cancer Journal for Clinicians **22**:284-291, 1972.
3. Ruben, H. L.: Family crises, American Family Physician **11**:132-136, Feb., 1975.
4. Solzhenitsyn, A.: Cancer ward, New York, 1969, Farrar, Straus & Giroux, Inc.

16 Cancer Lifeline

a community-based crisis intervention service for cancer patients and their loved ones

JOYCE ANN HARLEY DOAN

Drop the cursed pettiness that belongs to men that live their lives as
if death will never touch them.

Don Juan

"My friend has cancer. What do I say when I visit?" "Is it okay to talk
about 'it'?" "Do other people with cancer feel this way?" Such questions are
common among callers in their conversations with Cancer Lifeline volunteers.
Cancer Lifeline, Inc., of Seattle, Washington, has been functioning as a special
service for persons facing cancer since March, 1974. Its major goal has been to
meet some of the emotional needs of people with cancer as well as their loved
ones. The purpose of this chapter is (1) to review briefly the philosophic, sociologic, and psychologic considerations that have guided the development of Cancer
Lifeline; (2) to describe the development of a functional program; (3) to summarize what has been learned during the first year of operation; and (4) to state
some implications such a service has for the nursing profession.

THEORETIC CONSIDERATIONS
Philosophic issues

Today the existential problem of finding meaning in one's own living and dying
is often complicated by loss of identity with a singular culture. For most Americans there is no unchanging, uniform sociocultural environment that at once offers
reasons for the coexisting forces of reality and teaches a way of coping with
them. Instead, modern man is confused by the paradoxes of love and hate, creation and destruction, and life and death, and often responds with a denial that
leaves him anxious and unprepared in the face of his own negative instincts.
Frankl[4] observed that in the absence of a stable social tradition, many people
experience an "existential vacuum." For one person this vacuum may stimulate a
creative search for personal meaning and fulfillment, whereas for another it leads
to a state of vacillation between boredom and overwhelming anxiety. The person

189

who chooses to engage in life and risks loving is more aware of loss and is more vulnerable to death. Again the paradox strikes: "Love is not only enriched by our sense of mortality but constituted by it."[10] Such a philosophic orientation speaks against the death-denying tendencies predominant in the last 50 years of American middle-class culture. Perhaps dying would be less of a disorienting crisis were people enabled to integrate it into their own world view at an earlier age.

Sociologic issues

Sociologists and anthropologists have approached the problems of life and death in a different way. They see most Americans experiencing the grief and loss caused by moving away from home, family, and friends. In addition to the stress of increased mobility, sociologists have cited constant social change, impersonal services aimed at capitalistic gain, and faith in technology as stressful, demoralizing forces in the American's everyday experience. Relationships in which there is nurturing, warm, personal caring are idealized but seldom realized in the restless mood of change.

Weiss[14] has identified six specific kinds of relationships necessary for individual well-being. One of them is a person's need for assurance of assistance in times of trouble. At one time extended family members offered this form of security, but because very few people still have easy accessibility to relatives beyond the nuclear family, such security is not available to many Americans. In the face of a life-threatening illness, death, and dying, the person may well have reason to fear isolation and loneliness. It is the fortunate individual who has cultivated friends who are able to become a substitute family in times of crisis. The fact that Threshold, in Los Angeles, has made a business of providing "death companions" for $7.50 an hour to comfort the dying is a real statement about American culture.[2] When a business must be established to care for another's most basic human needs, the viability of the entire social system seems to be called into question.

A second sociologic issue hinged on the one just reviewed is the shift into "patienthood" imposed on and/or required of the dying person.[9] This forced dependence on the medical system both releases society from responsibility for the seriously ill person and creates for the physician a myth of omnipotence. The physician, however, is held accountable legally only for the management of the patient's physical needs and has little time or training to deal with emotional aspects of the illness.[7] In the past half century, dying in an institution rather than at home has become the norm because of the nuclear family's isolation, lack of a religious community to act as an extended family, and the physician's separateness from the secular community. Weisman[13] suggested that "the circumstances of 'patienthood' often contribute more to a dying person's incapacity, suffering and disorientation than does the specific disease itself." We as a society need to look at what constitutes a purposeful, dignified death instead of robbing it of meaning by insisting on reducing it strictly to medical issues.

Psychologic issues

Several authors in recent writings about death and dying have differentiated the problems of dying from those of death.[3,6] A person's death affects the lives of others, whereas his dying not only touches others but also creates uniquely personal problems. Cancer is no doubt the most dreaded of the major diseases in America. One would rarely *choose* to die of cancer, since it can mean prolonged physical pain and suffering as well as physical disability and deterioration. It may also mean financial distress due to many medical bills. Cancer can mean loss of control and independence, and it can create social and psychologic isolation if loved ones are afraid of the disease or of death. When cancer is a terminal condition, it usually leaves time for reflection on one's own accomplishments in life— and time for psychologic pain when there are regrets. Each of these problems can bring emotional distress to the seriously ill or dying person and needs to be handled in a genuine, caring manner.

DEVELOPING CANCER LIFELINE AS A FUNCTIONAL AGENCY

One of the purposes of this chapter is to describe the process of developing Cancer Lifeline. The reader should bear in mind that no two communities are identical in needs or in existing services. Therefore, the elements of process and objectives to be reviewed could be applied anywhere, but the methods of implementation will probably differ from one community to another.

Process

The first phase of development was begun by a woman who had experienced the psychologic trauma concomitant with breast cancer. Before her illness Mrs. G. had worked with a crisis clinic in Seattle that provides a 24-hour phone service for people in emotional distress. Experiencing fragmented care and minimal help with psychologic readjustments, she believed that there must be a way to provide emotional support specific to the needs of people facing cancer. Mrs. G. began to test the interests of various contacts in and out of the medical field. From these contacts emerged an advisory committee that provided the source for the first board of directors, as well as outlined the components deemed necessary for a viable, effective organization. The King's County Medical Association, the county and state American Cancer Society, the Crisis Clinic, and representatives of various hospitals gave input and support to the project. By September, 1973, a group of twenty people had committed themselves to be the first outreach volunteers of Cancer Lifeline. They designed a 20-hour training program with the help of their board and the Crisis Clinic staff. After training had been completed and sufficient plans for publicity made, the service opened March 1, 1974. When the story of Mrs. G.'s illness and her idea was carried in a major local newspaper in the month of March, it stimulated forty to fifty calls. This response affirmed the fact that many unmet needs existed, and the challenge became one of discerning which portion of those needs Cancer Lifeline could promise to help meet.

The next big hurdle was to secure sufficient monies to pay for a part-time clinical coordinator and various organizational expenses. The Crisis Clinic, a charter agency receiving United Way monies each year, agreed to sponsor Cancer Lifeline as a demonstration and development project of United Way. A small grant for this purpose was received in October, 1974, for 6 months, and a similar grant is presently being considered for another year. The American Cancer Society also responded to a request for development monies. Stipends for speaking and teaching engagements as well as miscellaneous small donations have helped with some of the expenses involved in getting a new organization started.

At the time that the monies for the United Way demonstration and development project became available, a clinical coordinator was hired. It was felt that a person with skills in counseling and nursing would be desirable. The present coordinator is a master's degree candidate in family nursing and was in the charter group of Cancer Lifeline outreach workers.

Objectives

Much of the rationale for the structure of Cancer Lifeline has been reviewed. The objectives and methods of implementation are as follows:

1. *To provide clients with immediate and continual accessibility to caring, helping individuals.* This goal was implemented in part by affiliating with a well-established 24-hour telephone service, the crisis clinic, for brief intake and screening. This has avoided duplication of direct 24-hour telephone coverage and allowed Cancer Lifeline's volunteers to respond to clients from their homes and in some cases their places of work. The following steps are involved in connecting an outreach worker with a client:

   a. The prospective client calls the Crisis Clinic and gives name, telephone number, and a brief statement about the nature and urgency of the problem.

   b. The Crisis Clinic telephone worker contacts the Cancer Lifeline volunteer on "first call."

   c. The Cancer Lifeline volunteer attempts to match the needs expressed by the client with the capabilities of several volunteers.

   d. One of these volunteers is contacted and agrees to return the client's call. This system has worked well enough to return a call within 5 to 10 minutes, if necessary.

Cancer Lifeline viewed the telephone contact as an effective vehicle for extending help but wanted to go beyond this point when the caller wished more personal contact. Therefore each volunteer is trained for home and hospital visitation as well. The organization was aware that no other agency offered emotional support as its primary objective in providing services for cancer patients and their loved ones. Yet, as has been reviewed, emotional support appears critical to the positive adjustment of many persons facing cancer. "Outreach" workers have provided some direct support to cancer patients as well as elicited more effective support from family members and friends. In some cases referral to other resources is indicated. The one rule followed diligently is that clients initiate almost all contacts unless they have specifically requested regular follow-up.

2. *To maintain and improve the quality of services offered by Cancer Lifeline.* The key to providing consistent, sensitive outreach services lies in the combination of screening and training the volunteer. Each volunteer is expected to attend 20 hours of training prior to receiving any calls and is then asked to commit several hours each month to in-service meetings. Even volunteers who have had formal education in counseling, nursing, or other helping professions attend training in order to be oriented to the basic philosophy and structure of Cancer Lifeline. The following areas are covered in the training program:

  a. Cancer in its medical context, including the function and importance of the doctor-patient relationship
  b. Grief and loss, death and dying, as they affect the person with terminal cancer, the person's loved ones, *and* the volunteer
  c. Theory and practice of crisis intervention by telephone and in person
  d. Role playing with various situations that commonly arise in calls and visits

Logs and standardized record keeping of each call provide data that can be reviewed and assessed at any time. When the outreach worker completes a call or visit, important content is recorded and sent to the clinical coordinator. The last heading of the record form is "Evaluation of the Contact," which is meant to encourage the volunteer to think critically about the quality of the interaction with the client.

3. *To explore alternative methods for providing client support.* This objective was one of the longer-range goals for the organization. From January through March, 1975, the clinical coordinator of Cancer Lifeline joined with a social worker from a United Way–subsidized counseling service in co-leading a group for women who had undergone surgery for breast cancer. This group was formed, as an extension of Cancer Lifeline, of women with mastectomies, to deal with self-image and body loss, femaleness, fear and anger about cancer, death and dying, and problems in communicating with those who are close. This opportunity was used to look critically at what a group might offer that would differ from one-to-one contact. The intent of the organization is to be supportive of any group experiences for cancer patients and their families when qualified leadership is demonstrated. Direct sponsorship of groups will occur when there are sufficient financial and staff resources to make it possible.

4. *To respond to and act on community feedback.* As a project seeking to help with unmet needs, Cancer Lifeline has defined some of its parameters of activity as a result of input from clients and institutions needing its services. One open question has been how to maintain autonomy when viability eventually may depend on merging with a compatible, well-founded organization. The flexibility that has been the privilege of a new and separate agency has been a real asset.

However, inefficiency occurs when a relatively small group must use much of its budget to pay for headquarters, equipment, and secretarial help. It is hoped that in the coming year a parent organization will agree to help with operational costs while allowing Cancer Lifeline to remain semi-independent from the dictates of the parent board. At a time when the economy is curtailing many new and old service endeavors, it is a statement of faith to believe that Cancer Lifeline will be one agency the community continues to support.

RESPONSE DURING FIRST YEAR
Volunteer response

It is the rare individual who is not familiar with the psychologic impact of cancer either as a patient or as a friend or relative of one. Many health professionals realize that they are unable to provide adequate emotional support to those facing cancer because job descriptions and institutions limit time and flexibility. Society has often responded to gaps in various services by utilizing volunteers. A study published in 1972[8] found that today many volunteers are carefully selected and take responsibility for highly sensitive helping roles. Another author, Conley, concluded that some services initially provided by volunteers are a major stimulus for improving care in long-established agencies and institutions.[8]

Cancer Lifeline screens its volunteers by telephone or personal interviews, a pretraining application, and observation of the individual during training. Volunteers have brought a variety of skills and experiences into the organization. Some are nurses, others have social work or counseling backgrounds, some have had cancer and wish to help others, some have lost a spouse or family member, and still others realize they are good listeners and have empathy for those facing serious illness. Turnover because of moves, changes in job status, or need for a rest has affected five of the sixteen charter outreach volunteers. Two training groups since the first in September, 1973, give Cancer Lifeline a present capacity of thirty outreach workers. This number maintains the desired ratio of one volunteer for every two clients per month. Such a ratio increases the likelihood of matching the volunteer's age, experiences, and needs with those of the client, as well as keeps any one volunteer from becoming overworked. Five volunteers have had cancer, four are men, and five are women who have lost husbands with cancer. The remainder have cared for family members with cancer or work with cancer patients in a professional capacity. The greatest problem to date has been finding volunteers with free time during the day to make calls.

Client response

The number of requests for help has varied from month to month and seems to be contingent in part on the amount and type of publicity. Newspaper articles stimulate more calls than periodic radio and television advertisements. Cancer Lifeline is currently averaging one new client a day.

It was expected that many callers would want personal contact with the outreach worker. To date, only 15% of the clients have asked for visits at some point. Distance has prohibited visits in only a few instances. Most often the caller will initiate contact at a point of crisis and discontinues the telephone conversation in 30 to 60 minutes. Sixty percent of the callers have telephoned only once. These people indicate that they have family, friends, and health care professionals from whom they usually receive support. When they fear that they have overburdened these people or are uncertain about who can help with a new problem, they may then call on Cancer Lifeline.

Another plausible explanation for telephone contact as the preferred mode of support is that 85% of the clients are women. At the risk of making sexist generalizations, empirical observation suggests that the American woman has learned to use the telephone very differently from men in this country. Women seem more able to share personal matters with friends by telephone (and in person). Having cultivated telephone conversations as meaningful contact, women appear better able to use the telephone with helping individuals in times of crisis. Other factors that may make telephone contact more acceptable to the client are the ease with which the caller can control the interaction, the fact that fewer pressures are on the caller to look and be his or her "best," and the possibility of obtaining immediate assistance without inconveniencing the client or the outreach worker.

Approximately 15% of the clients have had personal visits with outreach workers. Home or hospital visits are made when long-term contact with the client is anticipated, when the client's family needs to be involved in the crisis or problem resolution, and when the client expresses great loneliness. When the client asks for intervention involving the entire family, a team of two volunteers make the home visit together. Usually the family is having trouble talking openly about cancer and/or impending death. Two volunteers can help each other when family "games" occur or feelings become intense. The situation is especially tense when a mother is dying of cancer and has children still dependent on her. The stormiest problems have occurred with teenagers who find the normal identity crisis of adolescence heightened by the threatened or actual loss of a parent.[5]

Sixty percent of Cancer Lifeline's clients call about a friend or relative with cancer, and the other 40% call about themselves. Of this latter group, 34% have had breast cancer, and nearly three fourths of all those with cancer were experiencing a recurrence or the terminal phase of their disease. The age curve began in the 20s, peaked at 40 to 60 years of age, and then fell abruptly. Three fourths of those calling about themselves wanted to talk about feelings related to cancer, death, and dying. One fourth of this group had some questions and/or complaints about their medical care, with one third needing to clarify their own feelings about treatment. Twelve percent of this group mentioned thoughts of suicide, usually in a philosophic way. People with cancer need to learn what is normal "illness behavior" for persons facing this disease. Many clients have wondered aloud about their reactions of anger, depression, fear, and various treatment-related experiences.

Among the persons who called about loved ones, 22% were concerned about a spouse, 44% about some other family member, and 33% about a friend. Feelings about cancer, death, and dying were discussed by 40% of this group, as were questions about what to say to the person with cancer. Twenty percent were trying to decide whether home, hospital, or nursing home care was best for the person with cancer, 15% asked for various kinds of medical information (and were especially curious about the unproved cancer "cure" Laetrile), and 10% of family and friends wanted to know about financial resources.

An evaluation of effectiveness (beyond the self-critique made by the volunteer on the report form) is just being started. Every fifth caller will be contacted a month or more from the last contact and asked some form questions. Responses to date have been very positive. The greatest resistance tends to occur with clients who ask to talk with someone who has had their type of cancer and/or treatment.

Community response

Beyond the community's acceptance of Cancer Lifeline as a legitimate and qualified service, various other helping programs have turned to Cancer Lifeline for input. Some have wanted instruction in how to approach and assist persons facing serious illness and death. Several hospitals have wanted to learn specifically about Cancer Lifeline and how to use its services appropriately. Professional groups have asked for Cancer Lifeline representation in discussions and planning for better delivery of care to persons with cancer and other life-threatening illnesses. The American Cancer Society has maintained a reciprocal relationship with Cancer Lifeline, offering specific kinds of aid in return for help with certain clients and training of its own volunteers. The challenge of the requests from various community groups is knowing how to meet these requests without jeopardizing or compromising personal service.

IMPLICATIONS FOR NURSING SERVICES

Cancer Lifeline, Inc., of Seattle, Washington, offers assistance to persons experiencing the emotional distress of cancer, death, and dying. Since March, 1974, the project has been increasingly utilized by persons with cancer and by their loved ones. It is supported by established agencies and institutions that meet other needs of cancer patients and is expanded by continuing volunteer help. As medical knowledge increases and demands specialization, the cancer patient often experiences fragmented care and confusion about who will care for such primary needs as psychologic and emotional support. Some people who have turned to Cancer Lifeline needed help in using the medical system more effectively. Others needed to know whether their reactions constituted "normal illness behavior," whereas loved ones wanted help in understanding and coping with this behavior. Some needed to talk with an objective party about feelings of loneliness, fear, despair, guilt, and anger.

Some health professionals have questioned the ability of volunteers to meet such sensitive aspects of care. Anderson suggested that professionals have more difficulty with the idea of lay help than do patients, because institutional structure is vertical, with professionals at the top as helpers and the lay person in the position of need.[8] As was indicated, Cancer Lifeline's volunteer population includes professionals who know the deficiencies of their own work situations and lay persons who know they have something special to give. The success of Cancer Lifeline has been due in part to the range of abilities volunteers have brought to the organization and shared with each other. Nurses involved in the program have found it a satisfying way to participate in the community as well as to expand their education.

The advent of Cancer Lifeline should jolt the complacency of health care professionals in their belief that much patient care is left undone because it is financially prohibitive. This belief can become a convenient excuse for avoiding anxiety-laden issues of patient care. Through friends, Cancer Lifeline became operational within 6 months from the first meeting of the advisory committee. Few professionals could claim such rapid advances in their own program planning.

One social change that has affected nurses and physicians in the last decade is the popularity of a previously taboo subject—death and dying. Feifel and Kübler-Ross have been pioneers in formulating theoretic frameworks for understanding this experience that is part of each person's life. One of the hazards of theory has always been its use as a defense instead of as a vehicle to understanding and growth. A poignant reminder of the misuse of present theory by health professionals is found in the poetry of a man dying of leukemia. Ted Rosenthal wrote in *How Could I Not Be Among You?**:

> All those people who say that you are predictable and that you will die in the same way that everyone else dies, they are right. I resented that at first. I resented them saying "Oh you are at the two week stage. You're feeling, doing this. You're free. You're at the angry stage. I understand that. You're depressed. You're lost. Three and one half weeks after you find this out you always feel lost."
> Well, they're right. It works that way with me. I am following patterns. I am following the guidelines for dying-of-terminal-cancer-patients down to the letter. They all told me how this would be, how I would be reacting. It's fiendish. No matter what I say, they say, "Hm. That's what we thought you'd say." Especially the nurses—and the doctors, too. All of them.

How often professionals substitute a diagnosis for a solution to the patient's problem, when it is more likely a solution to their own.

Nurses need, too, to make themselves more available to cancer patients and their families. Few callers have mentioned an office or hospital nurse as the per-

---

*From Rosenthal, Ted: How could I not be among you, New York, 1973, George Braziller, Inc. Copyright 1973 by Ted Rosenthal.

son chosen for emotional support in the medical system. In a study reviewed in *The New England Journal of Medicine*[11] twenty-six families caring for loved ones at home indicated that they had many expectations of physicians, including psychologic support, whereas home nursing services were neither mentioned nor used. Nurses may complain that physicians or confining job descriptions hold them back from doing what they would like to do for cancer patients. Although this is true in part, it is time for the profession to become less tolerant of prescribed roles if nurses believe that the patient suffers because of the present status of health-care delivery.

A final point is made as a reminder that being a professional is not synonymous with being able to face death. The question is often asked, "How do people approach their own death?" The obvious reply after a year of conversations with persons at various places on the dying continuum is that people face death much as they face life. Persons with cancer have shown that the best preparation for dying is to live each day in such a way that life would feel complete if death should "tap them on the shoulder."

REFERENCES

1. Castaneda, C.: Journey to Ixtlan: the lessons of Don Juan, New York, 1973, Simon & Schuster, Inc., p. 56.
2. Death companionship, Time, Feb. 17, 1975, p. 68.
3. Dumont, R. G., and Foss, D. C.: The American view of death: acceptance or denial? Cambridge, Mass., 1972, Schenkman Publishing Co., Inc.
4. Frankl, V.: Man's search for meaning, New York, 1963, Washington Square Press, Inc.
5. Hansburg, H. G.: Adolescent separation anxiety, Springfield, Ill., 1973, Charles C Thomas, Publisher.
6. Hinton, J.: Dying, Baltimore, 1967, Penguin Books, Inc.
7. Klagsbrun, S. C.: Communications in the treatment of cancer, The American Journal of Nursing 71:944, May, 1971.
8. Knowledge Utilization Conference on the Use of Volunteers in Vocational Rehabilitation and Public Welfare Agencies: Volunteers for people in need, Washington, D.C., Nov., 1972, Department of Health, Education, and Welfare.
9. Krant, M.: In the context of dying. In Schoenberg, B., and others: Psychological aspects of terminal care, New York, 1972, Columbia University Press.
10. May, R.: Love and will, New York, 1969, Dell Publishing Co., Inc., p. 101.
11. Rose, M. A.: Help for the cancer patient's family, The New England Journal of Medicine 292:433, Feb. 20, 1975.
12. Rosenthal, T.: How could I not be among you? New York, 1973, George Braziller, Inc., pp. 24-25.
13. Weisman, A. T.: On death and denying, New York, 1972, Behavioral Publications, Inc., p. 33.
14. Weiss, R. S.: The fund of sociability, Trans-Action 10:36, Aug., 1969.

ADDITIONAL READINGS

Feifel, H., editor: The meaning of death, New York, 1959, McGraw-Hill Book Co.
Kübler-Ross, E.: On death and dying, New York, 1969, The Macmillan Co.
Solzhenitsyn, A.: Cancer ward, New York, 1969, Bantam Books, Inc.

17 Terminal illness at home
coordination of care and comfort

P. M. MacELVEEN

Management of terminal illness at home is a multifaceted challenge for the nurse. Although the patient's needs remain central, other important concerns emerge within the context of this situation: persons are likely to require teaching and support to fulfill their care-giving efforts; individual and family needs cannot be ignored; and mobilization of patient, family, and community resources and of network support systems is often critical for long-term home care situations. Opportunities for primary prevention assessments and interventions are numerous as the patient and family deal with the intense dynamics associated with death and dying.

The concerns expressed here will revolve around the terminal stage of illness— the patient's dying. These terms are difficult to define precisely and are used interchangeably. *Terminally ill* and *dying* refer to the time when alternative efforts to combat the progress of the disease are exhausted, or the patient declines further treatment; the patient is no longer able to fulfill usual family, occupational, and social roles, and inherent in the patient's progressive deterioration are the increased limitations in function and independence.

At this point, there is an appropriate shift of goals from the pursuit of cure to the provision of care, comfort, and a dignified death. Achievement of these latter goals does not come by passively yielding to the inevitable death. On the contrary, aggressive efforts are made to maintain the optimal function available for the patient for as long as possible; to assist the patient and family to maximize the living time they have left to share; and to help all involved to participate in a peaceful death for the patient.

Nurses in public health agencies, visiting nurse services, and some oncology units are assisting those families involved in home care of terminally ill members. However, the American literature addressing the issues of home care of the dying found by this author focused on only a few accounts of personal experiences by nurses involved in the management of terminal care for a relative or friend.[2,4,9] Reports from a British symposium on the care of the dying, held by the Royal College of Surgeons in 1972, estimated that more than one third of those persons dying of cancer are cared for at home. Lay persons, physicians, nurses, and social workers shared their concerns, knowledge, and experiences about terminal care in a joint effort to improve the standards of care of the dying. Much attention was

199

expressed about the needs of both patient and family. The renowned St. Christopher's Hospice, in London, which offers dedicated care to the dying, has continued to expand the home services program, which supports dying patients who remain at home and their families.[10] Dying at the hospice is seen as the next best place to dying at home when good care is not available there.

In some situations, institutional care is necessary for medical, social, or psychologic reasons. However, where specialized care will not add greatly to the length or quality of life, the patient may want to spend his last days amid the people he loves. Imposed separation in these circumstances is tragic. Why, then, do so few people die at home?

INSTITUTIONALIZATION OF DYING

Numerous changes in society have influenced where terminal care will be given. During the twentieth century, increasing control over life and death has resulted from the exponential development of medical knowledge and biomedical technology. Such medical progress could not be incorporated into the physician's office but required money, space, technicians, and other resources for availability. Thus the hospital became the workshop of the physician. Management of the very sick shifted from the patient's home to the hospital. As more sick patients were hospitalized, nurses who had previously practiced in patients' homes followed their clients into the hospitals.

Family life has also undergone much change in this century. Modern American families rarely include three generations or unmarried adult women in a household; relatives are frequently separated by geographic or social distance. In the past, the women at home looked after ill members of their households. With the changing status of women and changing economic values, many women work outside the home, so that countless homes are empty during the daytime. No one is there who can give care for illness that lasts more than a few days. Private insurance and Medicare have contributed their influence to moving the dying person out of the home. Most insurance coverage has no provision for care services to be delivered to the patient who is terminally ill at home. Therefore, when care can no longer be managed at home, the patient is transferred to a hospital or nursing home.

During the last 30 years, the number of deaths occurring in institutions has doubled, and currently about two thirds of all deaths occur in hospitals or nursing homes.[8] One might assume that the staff members dealing so frequently with death would become specialists or experts. Findings from studies on death and dying by researchers from a variety of disciplines indicate otherwise. Benoliel,[1] Glaser and Strauss,[5] Kübler-Ross,[7] and Sudnow[11] agree that dying, one of the most singular events in the human experience, is often endured by patients as an artificially prolonged, dehumanizing agony in an atmosphere of abandonment and profound loneliness.

Science, which has freed man from many of the consequences of ignorance and superstition, has thus far failed to provide satisfying understandings of the meaning of life and death. Modern man fears his own mortality no less than his ancestors did. The efforts to deny death are manifest in the prolongation of dying and the greater sufferings of the patient.

DYING AT HOME

The comfortable familiarity of one's own home and bed becomes increasingly important when one is frightened, sick, aged, or dying. The sights, sounds, smells, feelings, and even the vibrations as the furnace clicks on are known and understandable. Personal possessions are memory banks of people and events from other days. There is an ease in knowing how to go from the bed to the bathroom, and where doorways and furniture are if there is a need to hold on for a minute.

When the patient has established satisfying relationships within the family, the family members know the little things that are significant, even if they might seem amusing to someone else. Time, which becomes a very precious commodity to the patient who is terminally ill, may be spent sharing stories about old times, putting affairs in order, watching a white rose unfold, or just quietly being near loved ones.

Even in the terminal stage, the woman with a husband and children can share much of the family life by simply being there at home with them, even though she is not able to actively fulfill her roles. Her children are not left to create fearful fantasies to explain her death, when they have been able to be with her as her strength fades. Family life is not disrupted by the father's absence, as it is when he frequently goes to visit mother in the hospital, where the children may not be allowed to enter. Indeed, unless the hospital or nursing home is conveniently close by, the time spent traveling, visiting, waiting, and so on, may be extremely fatiguing.

Some families may welcome the opportunity to take care of the patient at home, trusting that their physician believes they can do so, and that they will be helped to accomplish whatever needs to be done. Most often, a mother, wife, sister, or other woman in the family takes on the major responsibility for care. Occasionally, when no relative is available, a woman may emerge from the friendship network who is willing to assist the family.

Other families may wish that they could respond to the patient's desires but may not have anyone available who is both comfortable in giving care and able to do so. In the case of an older couple, the spouse may also be in poor health or may not be strong enough to give care if the patient becomes bedridden. Home care may not be possible in these situations unless help emerges from the social network of friends or relatives.

Still other families may want very much to care for the patient at home but are not sure how they could manage. All the families need help in identifying the predictable care needs, what resources they could mobilize within their own social network, and what community resources are available to them. Caring for the dying person impinges on all the members of the family, directly or indirectly.

Depending on the duration of the illness and any special care needs, some temporary adjustments of family life are likely to be necessary.

The patterns and quality of most relationships within the family system are not likely to change at the terminal stage of the patient's illness. Relatives may have limits to the time and energy they are willing to allocate to the care of the dying person. In this case, although the patient remains at home, it is unlikely that the care and comfort needed will be given. Transfer to a nursing home might be a welcome alternative.

Investment in the caring procedures, the high fidelity of interactions if there is a shared awareness of the dying, and the family's participation together can result in an extremely valuable experience. Mrs. B's pancreatic carcinoma had widely metastasized at the time of diagnosis. She rejected the offer of chemotherapy and understood that she probably had less than a year to live. Within a few days of this unexpected event, Mrs. B., still somewhat in a state of shock and disbelief, said: "You know, there's a freedom in knowing that you are dying. You don't have to pretend any more. There's no need to try to be anything except what I really am. It's like a burden being lifted off my shoulders."

A rich degree of intimacy and communication is available in the relationship with a patient who shares openly the knowledge that death is near. After the death, families who provided terminal care often have satisfying feelings about fulfilling the patient's desire to die at home. Wolfle[13] found that during the year following a death, the mortality rate was twice as high in families whose relative had died in a hospital or nursing home as among families whose relative had died at home.

Participatory planning and decision making

How does the decision to die at home come about? Sometimes the patient or relative simply asks the physician whether the care can be given at home. However, many people have no experience with dying and no idea what care might be necessary. They may not know that the wants of the terminally ill are usually quite simple: to be free from intolerable pain, to be near the people they love, and not to be alone when they die. In most cases, these needs are easily met at home if the patient has people who are willing and able to give care. When the family steadfastly refuses to consider home care, even with the assurance of support, the patient must seek other alternatives.

If the nurse is to coordinate the care with the patient and family at home, she becomes the liaison between them and the services they may need. Depending on the patient's situation, the nurse may be in contact with the physician, hospital personnel, social worker, clergyman, home health aid, etc.

Ideally, if the patient and family share the information of the patient's prognosis, then determination of the management of home care can be achieved by patient, family, nurse, and physician together. Planning can be shared, and the agreement, or contract, may be that the patient be cared for at home as long as it is possible to give good care there. This agreement allows for alternative planning at some later time if there are changes in the patient's needs, in the ability of the family to endure over a long period of time, or in the health status of family members, or if there are other problems reducing the effectiveness of home care. If the patient continues to use denial, that need is respected, and tentative plans may be made without the patient until he is ready to be included.

Participation in the planning and decision making is significant for another important reason. Inclusion of patients recognizes their personhood and their right to determine, to whatever extent possible, what will happen to them. As their physical limitations increase and their sphere of control shrinks, feelings of helplessness, powerlessness, and dependency may be more difficult to bear than physical pain. When the patient no longer wants or needs to have control, the response to a needed decision is usually quite clear: "You take care of it. . . ."

Since the length of the terminal stage is not always predictable, the family is entering into an open-ended contract that may extend from a few weeks to many months. In order to provide good care, the family members must not feel trapped, and they must know that they will be supported in finding alternatives if the care situation exceeds their abilities or energy resources at any time. When the care is given for a period of time at home, and then the patient is moved to another setting, the patient is told that special care has become necessary. The family members are assured that they did give good care during the home care and permitted the patient to be at home as desired. In this way, they can be helped to feel that they have done their best.

A few physicians include support of the desire to die at home as part of their practice. Most often, the care is coordinated by a nurse from a community health agency. When the family is known to the nurse before the patient reaches the terminal stage, the nurse has an early opportunity to begin identifying family strengths and resources.

The following factors are critical considered in terminal care of the patient at home:

1. The kind of care likely to be required
2. The adaptability of the home environment to that care
3. The ability of family members in the home to deal with the patient's dying
4. The availability of one or two persons willing and able to give the care that is needed
5. The availability of a nurse (or another helping professional) to coordinate the home care

The family's assessment of these factors may differ from the nurse's, and their assessment must be known if it is to be taken into account. For example, a woman with a small house willingly chose to turn the living room into a sickroom so that her dying husband will not be separated from her and their children. Discussion with patient, family, physician, and nurse on the above issues will determine the feasibility of terminal care at home. The nurse who has made a home visit contributes valuable data from assessments, especially concerning what equipment or services could enhance the home situation if the patient is to receive home care.

Assessment of needs

In the immediate period after the cessation of aggressive treatment at the hospital or clinic, the patient may make some physical gains if he is recuperating from a surgical procedure or radiation therapy. The nurse helps the patient and family to define reasonable goals for the patient. Together they work on a plan to achieve the goals, restoring as much well-being and function as might temporarily be available. The nurse teaches them how to carry out the interventions they agree help move the patient toward their shared goals.

The nurse has her own set of patient assessments, problem priorities, and interventions to be addressed. The patient and family will perceive the situation through their own needs. Congruency around goals and means to achieve goals is likely to be achieved among those involved with the patient's care as they share in the identification of problems and work together toward solutions. When patient-family-nurse goals, priorities, or means to goals are not immediately congruent or are in conflict, further discussion and reassessment are in order.

After an amputation of his right leg for a sarcoma, 70-year-old Mr. M. refused to do his exercises because they were tiring, and he said they gave him more pain. He had not been convinced that it was realistic to believe that he could be ambulatory and therefore would not participate in the exercise program. The nurse shared with Mr. M. again that the exercises were aimed at helping him to gain strength so that he could use a walker and be up and around again. Independence was very important to Mr. M., and his hope not be bound to bed or wheelchair was temporarily realized. He greatly enjoyed being able to walk around his garden that summer for several months before he became bedridden a few weeks prior to his death.

Of particular concern to the patient and the family is the fear of pain and other discomforts. If we expect the patient to trust us to maintain comfort "later," we must keep promises to help maintain comfort as much as possible in present distress. Hinton[6] reports that the terminal stage, when patient distress is greatest, is likely to be only a few days or weeks, rarely more than 3 months. In all but a few extreme cases, most pain and discomfort can be managed.[12] (See Chapter 14.)

Special care is required for the patient who has had a colostomy, urethrostomy, tracheostomy, gastrostomy, etc. The patient should be supported in managing his own care as much as possible. With good teaching, the nurse can assist the patient and family to be responsible and competent in these special care areas.

Modification of the physical environment may be necessary for the patient's safety and maintenance of independence for as long as possible. Loose rugs should be removed to prevent falls, and furniture should be arranged to be convenient for the patient's use and to avoid obstacles in pathways. The bathtub should have nonslip rubber strips or matting for the patient who continues to want tub baths or showers. Measures should be taken to ensure the weakening patient's safety in getting into and out of the tub. An elevated toilet seat may solve the still-ambulatory patient's problem of how to get up when leg muscles are no longer strong enough. Eventually, a bottle urinal and chair commode may be necessary. The hospital bed becomes essential when the patient begins to receive any considerable amount of care in bed. A bedside telephone is useful not only for receiving calls while in bed but also for emergency use if the patient is alone in the house at times. Whatever efforts are made to extend the independence and control of the patient, even for just a short time, reinforce a sense of self-worth and demonstrate caring and concern for the patient's ability to have some measure of control over his life.

Where the patient is located in the home may vary greatly. One patient was centered in the dining room so that he could be at least a participant-observer of family life. In another family the patient was "protected" from the noise of young children by use of a bedroom away from the family activity areas.

Although the nurse may view the family's arrangement as untenable, the primary responsibility is to support the dying patient and the family in their efforts to provide care, comfort, and a dignified death at home, if that is what the patient chooses.

The training in the highly technologic procedures of hemodialysis in cases of end-stage renal failure is an excellent example of the potential of lay persons for self-care within the home. The transfer of the responsibility for treatment procedures from the professional nurse to the lay person is related to the shift in the nurse's role. This role is not diminished by such a change, but it is altered because these patients and families develop needs that are generated by the home dialysis situation. Teaching becomes a major task, along with supporting the use of coping skills by which the entire family maintains a healthy, growth-promoting system.

Similarly for the nurse coordinating terminal care, the psychosocial needs of the patient and the family are of major concern. These needs become increasingly critical as the time of death nears. Attention and energy tends to focus more and more on the patient. The grieving process begins for some family members before the death occurs, and at one level, they turn inward on their own experience. The nurse may facilitate the communications between the patient and those whom he leaves behind. The ability to share and talk together is important for the other members of the family during this time and during the grieving process after the death.

There is pain also as the patient attempts to absorb the meaning of his death. This process has been described at length by Kübler-Ross[7] as one in which the patient moves from shock and denial, through anger, bargaining, and depression, to the acceptance of his own death. The patient experiences a profound set of losses in letting go of almost everything of meaning and value: abilities, skills, and talents; cherished activities and experiences; independence, power, and control; body image; future plans, dreams, and aspirations; and, in the end, each loved person.

Disfiguring changes in the body and loss of weight and strength are very difficult for many patients. Mrs. K.'s inoperable tumor grew rapidly, and she referred to her greatly enlarged abdomen as being "not me." She avoided mirrors as her loss of weight became more and more apparent. When one day she allowed herself to look in the bathroom mirror, she was visibly shocked and shaken by her appearance. She wanted to stop visitors because she did not want people to see her looking so awful. She was encouraged to talk about her reactions to the changes she had observed. After several such discussions, she requested that a towel be hung over the bathroom mirror, and she again allowed some of her closer friends to visit.

During the period of terminal care, the family must cope with the patient's dying and yet continue the business of living. It is important that the needs of individual members be recognized and some means for meeting those needs defined. Family systems differ considerably according to their location in the life cycle. The retired husband looking after his dying wife with the help of an adult daughter who lives nearby is in quite a different situation from the woman with teenage children giving terminal care at home to her husband. The needs of a young family when the mother is dying, and neighbors and friends are helping the husband to care for her and the small children, create different problems.

The nurse must maintain an awareness of all the family members and how they are experiencing the current situation at home. Their ability not only to cope with the crisis but to meet other needs must be assessed. The more concern that is directed toward the dying person, the greater is the likelihood that other family members' psychosocial needs may not be met from within the system. There are families who become "exhausted" before the ordeal is over. This exhaustion results not only from extreme physical fatigue but also from the prolonged period during which individual family members do not have the means of meeting their own personal needs. When the family reaches this state, the desire to "get it over with" often generates feelings of resentment toward the dying person, as well as guilt for feeling that way. These feelings add to the burdens of the grieving process.

Identification of resources

Assessment of the home care situation implies the identification of patient and family strengths and resources. Being in crises together may elicit a cooperative spirit and cohesiveness. Families with a strong religious orientation derive much strength from their faith and the support of their clergy. Talking to the family together helps the nurse to assess communication and problem-solving skills.

As the time approaches when the patient will require increasing amounts of care or cannot be left alone, the family is alerted. Persons may emerge in the kinship network from nearby or come from a distance to help. Persons from the neighborhood, church, or friendship network may make themselves available. Some family member may have health care experience as a paraprofessional. A teenager's obvious caring relationship with a dying grandparent may indicate that he could help with some of the care, thereby relieving his mother occasionally.

Resources available in the kinship and friendship networks are many and varied, especially where these networks are characterized by reciprocity and intimacy. Some friends and relatives may give of their time, visiting and assisting with care of the patient, helping with shopping, babysitting, chauffeuring children, and giving spiritual and emotional support. Often the nurse can help the family members utilize these resources by helping them define discrete tasks appropriate to the offer to help. For example, a neighbor might come once a week on a regular basis for an hour and a half. This time might be used for errands, shopping, a trip to the library, or lunch with a friend.

Some nuclear families seem to have a rugged, independent style that prevents them from reaching out to kinship or friendship networks for assistance. These families are at greater risk during the prolonged crisis periods. They may, however, be able to utilize support from the nurse, physician, social worker, or clergyman.

In many communities a variety of groups and organizations respond to particular needs of patients with cancer, such as supplying of dressings, equipment, and emotional support to patients, their families, or friends. Local health care services may include the availability of home health aides, nurses' aides, and practical nurses. If these services are needed 8 hours a day, however, the costs may be almost as much as full care in a nursing home.

Designing the care plan

Involvement of the family and patient in problem solving and planning has already been discussed. The nurse's special knowledge and skills are valuable to all, since she is often able to anticipate needs, as well as help the patient and family to understand and respond to changes in the patient's condition. Nursing care efforts are likely to be focused on (1) maintenance of the patient's independence and maximal function for as long as possible; (2) management of distressing symptoms, especially pain; (3) support of the patient as he deals with his own dying; (4) modification of the environment to provide safety; and (5) inclusion of the patient in the family as far as possible.

These efforts relate to direct patient care and are familiar to nurses. Other efforts that focus on the family are significant, in that support of family members makes it possible for them to provide better care for the patient. The monitoring of family dynamics, reactions to the dying person, and anticipatory grieving are nursing efforts of primary prevention aimed at the family's physical and mental health.

When the patient's care is extensive, requires much time, or is likely to be protracted, the family may benefit from an organized division of labor, incorporating the offers of friends and relatives. The nurse can assist in the regular scheduling of some time out of the situation for the primary care giver, and of special times for the maintenance of husband-wife and parent-child relationships, which might otherwise be neglected. When care must be given over a period of several months, individual family members may need reassurance and legitimation from the nurse to meet such normal needs as sex, time alone, and recreation. Direction of all attention toward the dying person, to the exclusion of others, may occur prematurely, since families usually have little experience in anticipating when death might be imminent. The family's requests for information and support are likely to increase with time. Often they contact the nurse by phone for reassurance that they are doing the right thing, or for directions on how to respond to a new problem. The ability to contact the nurse or another helping person is important if the family is to feel secure that help is available when it is needed.

In the confrontation with death, or when death threatens a significant other, some persons have a strong urge to have sexual intercourse. Both men and women report this reaction. Perhaps, in a sense, intercourse is a reaffirmation of life in the face of death, or it may be that the closeness of death reaches into our existential loneliness and fear of death. Asking for sex may be easier than just asking to be held so as not to feel so alone.

A young couple who had lost an only child in a fatal accident confided that they had made love several times within the week of their infant son's death. "We felt so awful we just had to love each other." If the sexual urge is not mutual, a wife, for example, may misunderstand her husband's need for sex as insensitive, selfish, and inappropriate. Given the gravity of the situation defined by death, such an event might remain significant for a long period: his great need, unmet or unwillingly met; her hurt and indignation at his request.

When death does become imminent, families who have provided good care sometimes ask for the patient to be removed to a hospital for the final event of death. Perhaps they have a fearful fantasy about what actually will occur. There may be unspoken discomfort about somehow not knowing "the right things to do," which reflects the grim and mysterious notions about dead bodies common to our culture. Preparation of the family members for what they may observe happening to the patient at the time of death can reduce their fears. Explicit instructions about what to do after death are very important and comforting to the family. They would be planned to fit the specific family's needs, and might include, for example (1) call me; (2) call the physician; (3) call the funeral home; (4) wash the body with warm water; and (5) bring members of the family in who would like to say their good-byes. Such instructions assure the family that care at the time of death is not complicated and that they are competent to provide it.

Preparation for the patient's death also includes preparation for the period after death, when the family reconstitutes its dynamics and patterns without the patient. When possible, a follow-up visit several weeks after the death affords the nurse the opportunity to see how the family is managing and to terminate her relationship with them.

SUMMARY OF NURSING RESPONSIBILITIES

Coordination of home care for the terminally ill requires the nurse to have knowledge and understanding about the patient, the illness, the patient's family system, and community resources. The family system comes under the purview of the nurse during home visits especially. Making a continual assessment of the patient's changing care needs, teaching the care givers, supporting members of the family, and monitoring anticipatory grief and the family's tolerance for continuing terminal care are major nursing responsibilities.

Implicit in the approach described here is the inclusion of the patient and family in the planning and implementing of care, to the extent that they are able to participate. Sensitivity to changes in the patient and the family system may require modification of the care plan. Identification of strengths and resources of patient and family also includes their affiliations with a clergyman and congregation for spiritual and other supportive help. The potential resources among relatives, friends, and neighbors in their kinship and friendship networks can be very valuable. Mobilization of the latter is particularly important in prolonged situations.

Knowledge of the disease process, of dying and grieving, and of the use of self in a genuine relationship with the patient, and the willingness to risk involvement, are essential to the effectiveness of the nurse who works with the dying person at home.

REFERENCES

1. Benoliel, J. Q.: The practitioner's dilemma: problems and priorities. In Davis, R., editor: Confrontation with dying, Los Angeles, 1971, University of Southern California Press.
2. Blewett, L. J.: To die at home, American Journal of Nursing **70**:2602-2604, Dec., 1970.
3. Care of the Dying, British Medical Journal **3**:29-41, Jan., 1973.
4. Chura, V.: Sara wanted to die at home—but her family resisted, Nursing, 74, **4**: 16-18, July, 1974.
5. Glaser, B. G., and Strauss, A. L.: Awareness of dying, Chicago, 1965, Aldine Publishing Co.
6. Hinton, J.: Dying, Baltimore, 1967, Penguin Books, Inc.
7. Kübler-Ross, E.: On death and dying, New York 1969, The Macmillan Co.
8. Mushkin, S. J.: Consumer incentives for health care, New York, 1974, Prodist.
9. McNeil, D.: A death at home, The Canadian Nurse **70**:17-19, March, 1974.
10. McNulty, B. J.: St. Christopher's Outpatients, American Journal of Nursing **71**:2328-2330, Dec., 1971.
11. Sudnow, D.: Passing on, Englewood Cliffs, N.J., 1967, Prentice-Hall, Inc.
12. Twycross, R. G.: Principles and practices of the relief of pain in terminal cancer, Update, July, 1972.
13. Wolfle, D.: Dying with dignity, Science **168**:1403, June, 1970.

part V
REHABILITATION

The focus of the following two chapters is the rehabilitation of patients with cancer. Throughout this book we have presented chapters discussing the problem of awareness and the need to be open with the patient, the need for knowledge to develop a cancer consciousness and to screen or detect cancer early, the different approaches to therapy, and the need for maximizing the quality of life as it approaches termination. These two remaining chapters focus on the problems of rehabilitation—the problems of dealing with life while the disease process itself is in remission.

Ms. Saunders, in her chapter, looks at the problems faced by the patient who has gynecologic cancer. Once this disease is arrested or the patient experiences a remission, there are many questions that need to be answered so that these patients, as well as those patients with ongoing cancer, may regain a functional routine for management of day-to-day living.

Ms. Wear and Ms. Blessing look at the problems faced by the school-age child with leukemia. In their chapter they suggest ways to facilitate the child's return to school. From these authors' own experience, some specific forms have been devised to help not only the child but also the teacher, the parents, and the child's classmates in easing the child's return to the classroom once the disease is in remission.

In the final chapters of this book, we would like the reader to feel that, yes, cancer is a difficult disease to work with, but also that, yes, there is hope. Perhaps someday, as the periods of remission increase and the challenging problems of rehabilitation become more prevalent the quality of life for the cancer patient will be greatly enhanced. When these changes occur, we shall be able, as oncology nurses, to feel proud to have been a participant in the increasingly successful battle against an incurable disease.

ASSESSMENT FORM: GYNECOLOGIC CANCER

Name

Reproductive status

Age   Marital status

Number of children
Previous history of cancer in the family;
    in the patient
Age of menarche
Age of first pregnancy
History of fibrocystic breast disease
Onset of Menopause   Hormone therapy
Annual Pap smear
Previous surgical procedures or
    hospitalization
Understanding, feelings about illness

Ovarian and fallopian cancer   *Cancer of vagina*

Increase in abdominal girth   Mother given diethylstilbestrol (DES)
Lower abdominal discomfort   during pregnancy
Changing or fluctuating weight   Changes in vaginal discharge
Changes in menstrual cycle   Inguinal nodes
Inguinal nodes

Uterine cancer   *Cancer of vulva*

Changes in menstrual cycle   Persistent itching
Inguinal nodes   Inguinal or femoral lymph nodes

Assessment for patient undergoing abdominal radiation therapy

Skin   General
    Increased pigmentation   Leukopenia
    Protective clothing   Edema
    Flaking and itching   Thrombocytopenia
    Tenderness, delayed wound healing   Agranulocytosis
Gastrointestinal system
    Cramping
    Tenesmus
    Diarrhea
    Changes in electrolytes
    K+, Na+
    Nausea and vomiting

18 Considerations for rehabilitation for the patient with a gynecologic cancer

SAUNDRA ELAINE SAUNDERS

All patients with a diagnosis of cancer, whether there is a possibility for a cure or only for control of the disease, have certain needs in common that require careful attention from the professional health care team. Until life ceases, all patients have a life to live, knowledge to be gained, activities to do, responsibilities to fulfill, needs and desires to be answered, fears and frustrations to be alleviated, and the right to exercise as much control as possible over themselves and the actions taken in their behalf. The concept of rehabilitation—the returning of the patient to an optimum level of functioning—should be included in any plan of care for the patient with cancer, whether the patient has been cured of the disease or given only temporary control over that illness. In determining the extent of rehabilitation that is realistic for the patient, consideration must be taken of impending outcomes of the disease, whether cure or control is available, and what morbidity the patient may face from either the treatment or the disease itself.

Modern technology and research have given the health care team treatment modalities that, when used singly or in combination, have increased both the survival rates and cure rates for many cancers. It would seem that, with the improvement of methods of detection and public education, gynecologists now see far fewer patients with carcinoma of the cervix and subsequently fewer deaths. Combined radiation therapy and surgery have increased the survival rates for carcinoma of the uterus. A combination of surgery, chemotherapy, and radiation therapy has improved, to some extent, the outlook for the patient with a carcinoma of the ovary. Any one of these modalities, depending on the disease entity it is used to treat, and in the hands of a skilled clinician, can mean a cure for the patient involved. Cancer is still frightening and a horrible disease if unchecked. However, the outlook for the patient of today is far less grim than it was even one or two decades ago. Problems arise for the patient and the health care team when the disease is detected in its later stages, when previous treatment has been inadequate, and when there is morbidity arising from the treatment modalities themselves.

GYNECOLOGIC CANCERS, MODE OF TREATMENT, CURE RATES

The cancers that are treated in gynecology are discussed in this section in the order of their frequency. The treatments listed are those used at our institution and found in a technical bulletin produced by the American College of Obstetricians and Gynecologists in 1973.[3] Previously, the most commonly seen gynecologic can-

213

cer was carcinoma of the cervix, which, when discovered in the in situ stage, can be treated by either total abdominal hysterectomy or vaginal hysterectomy, with a 100% cure rate. If the patient is still of childbearing age and wishes to have children, treatment can be carried out with the use of conization that has all margins free of cancer and with careful follow-up of the patient. In its earlier stages carcinoma of the cervix is treated with radiation therapy in combination with a modified or radical hysterectomy, including node dissection. In later stages or when there is central recurrence, pelvic exenteration (which includes hysterectomy, vaginectomy, cystectomy with ileal conduit, and bowel resection with colostomy) is the treatment of choice. Radiation therapy (external and intracavitary) may be used for palliation; at present there is no chemotherapeutic drug that seems to be effective in control or cure of this disease. This cancer occurs in early adulthood and later, with the average age of development being 38 years.

Carcinoma of the ovary can be seen at any age but is seen predominantly from the age of 40 years. It is a dreaded disease because it is usually diagnosed at a later stage. The patient often presents herself to the physician after she has noticed an increase in abdominal girth with or without symptoms other than vague discomfort or fluctuating weight. The increased girth is caused by ascites, and at this time there is often extensive spread to other organs within the peritoneal cavity. Treatment is initiated with a total abdominal hysterectomy, bilateral salpingo-oophorectomy, partial omentectomy, and removal of all gross tumor. After the initial surgery, the patient may be returned for debulking of any persistent and growing tumor mass. Radiation therapy by abdominal bath or strip technique in which the upper abdomen is included, with a boosting dose to the pelvis, is used for the elimination of microscopic malignancy postoperatively. It is because tumor cells are more reactive to radiation therapy when the tumor mass is small that an attempt at debulking of the mass will almost always precede additional treatment for recurrent disease. Chemotherapy is used for palliation and is indicated in cases of malignant ascites, pleural effusion, massive residual tumor, distant metastasis, or radiation failure.

Carcinoma of the uterus or endometrium is usually seen in the postmenopausal woman. In the early stages of the disease, when it is treated by surgery alone or in combination with radiation therapy, the cure rate is around 90%. In later stages without metastasis, the cure rate is 70%, and with metastatic disease the cure rate drops to approximately 10%. Treatment for Stage 1 to Ia consists of total abdominal hysterectomy with a bilateral salpingo-oophorectomy. Stages Ib and II are treated by external and or internal (intracavitary) radiation therapy, followed in 4 to 6 weeks by a radical hysterectomy and pelvic lymph node dissection. Stage III is also treated by surgery and radiation therapy in either order, and in Stage IV, in cases in which the tumor is medically inoperable, chemotherapy is used for palliation.

Carcinoma of the vulva is a less frequently seen disease and is often initially mismanaged due in part to its infrequency, poor evaluation, and lack of biopsy, with subsequent inadequate treatment. It is found most often in the postmenopausal patient but can be found in younger women. One of its most frequent presenting symptoms is persistent itching of the vulva. The lymph system of the vulva is superficial, and early metastasis to the inguinal or femoral lymph nodes is common. A cure rate of 70% to 80% is found in those patients without lymph node metastasis. With involvement of the lymph nodes, survival falls to 40% to 50%. Survival rates for patients having deep pelvic lymph node metastasis are from 10% to 20%. Treatment of choice is by radical vulvectomy with pelvic lymphadenectomy. Radiation may be used for palliation in inoperable lesions to prevent extensive erosion and necrosis of tissue and provide comfort for the patient. Radiation therapy may also be used for palliation postoperatively in cases having positive lymph node pathology.

Carcinoma of the vagina is infrequently seen, having a cure rate of approximately 20% to 30%. In situ carcinomas of the vagina are treated with wide local excision of the lesion or by partial or total vaginectomy in some cases. Invasive carcinomas of the vagina are best treated by radiation therapy. Lesions found in the upper vagina may be a recurrence in patients previously treated for in situ carcinoma of the cervix. These lesions may be treated by radical excision of the lesion. It is important in detection of this malignancy that those women who have previously undergone hysterectomy be closely followed with routine pelvic examinations and Pap smears of the vaginal wall. There recently has been noted an increased incidence of clear-cell adenocarcinoma of the vagina in young women in their late teens and early twenties whose mothers were given diethylstilbestrol (DES) during pregnancy in an attempt to prevent a spontaneous abortion. At present it is believed that a cause-and-effect relationship cannot be definitely stated between these two occurrences, although information does point toward that possibility.

Carcinoma of the fallopian tube is the least commonly seen cancer of the reproductive system. Its symptoms are much like those seen in ovarian carcinoma, and the disease is frequently widespread on discovery. Current 5-year survival rates for this disease are 10% to 20%. Treatment is with total abdominal hysterectomy, bilateral salpingo-oophorectomy, and omentectomy, followed by total abdominal radiation therapy with a radiation boost to the pelvis. Palliation may result from the use of alkylating chemotherapeutic agents or multiple chemotherapeutic drugs.

HOW PATIENTS ARE CURED

When discussing "cure" for a patient with a gynecologic cancer, we are speaking of specific treatment modalities or combinations that include radiation therapy, surgery, radical surgery, a combination of radiation and surgery, and in rare instances, such as choriocarcinoma, chemotherapy. It should be noted that "radical surgery" is listed as a modality used for "cure," since it is felt by most cancer institutions that a patient should not undergo radical surgery and its inherent morbidity unless it is felt that there is a strong possibility of eradicating the disease, considering the involvement of that disease. The percentage of cure is small in those disease states in which radical surgery would be considered, such as middle to late stages, depending on the type of cancer involved, or in the case of a central recurrence in which other treatment modalities cannot be used. The physician needs to exercise careful consideration, evaluation, and judgment in determining the correctness of radical surgery in a particular situation. After the decision to offer radical surgery is made, it is important that careful attention be given to fully informing the patient as to what is hoped to be gained by the surgery, what changes in the patient can be expected as a result of the surgery, and what possible complications might be faced. The patient must then decide whether surgery will be performed or not. We have seen that patients will usually choose the surgery after being fully informed. Even if the patient should not choose to go through with the prescribed treatment, that patient should find total support from the health care team in the treatment and care of their subsequent health problems and needs.

The same concept of fully informing the patient holds true for the other treatment modalities as well. Patients should be aware that there are complications inherent in the different treatments available and should understand what those complications might mean to the patient's general health and well-being. The extent of information and the way it is imparted to the patient change somewhat with individual situations. However, all patients, to the limit of their capacity, should be fully informed of their treatment and its consequences. If the patient is informed, she is equipped to more quickly note impending problems and can then seek medical attention for such problems. She is also better equipped to plan for those activities in her life in which she either must be or wishes to be involved.

Radiation therapy

When patients receive radiation therapy for a gynecologic malignancy, the complications they face are those inherent in radiating as well the sensitive tissues of the bladder and bowel. Careful calculations made by a radiation physicist determine dosage that are tumoricidal to the cancer and yet relatively safe to the surrounding tissues. It has been found that normal cells can tolerate a certain amount of radiation, incurring only slight damage and maintaining the ability to heal and regenerate. The tumor cell, however, once it has been damaged, does not seem to be able to regenerate itself, but rather dies. It is this balance between a tumoricidal dose to the cancer and only a slightly damaging dose to surrounding tissues that is so important in preventing severe complications from the treatment. Records are kept so that treatments and their complication rates, in comparison to control and cure, can be studied over time in order to progress toward more definitive treatments with less frequent complications.

The complication seen most frequently with external radiation therapy is proctitis, which occurs with different degrees of severity. Careful checks are made in keeping track of gastrointestinal symptoms such as cramping, tenesmus, and diarrhea. Medication, usually Lomotil, is given for the control of diarrhea. However, if the symptoms persist, treatments are interrupted until the patient is returned to a more stable health status. This is done to prevent complications due to dehydration and electrolyte imbalance, which many patients, because of their advanced age and general debilitation, can reach in a very short period of time. Another reason for carefully following the patient's progress is the possibility of permanent damage to the bowel. Such damage can result in chronic proctitis or bleeding, or partial or complete bowel obstruction, which, if unable to be controlled medically, may lead to surgical intervention, with bowel resection and possibly an ostomy.

Other common side effects of radiation therapy to the abdomen as well as the pelvis are persistent nausea and vomiting or lack of appetite, which leads to dehydration as well as malnutrition and subsequent debilitation if left unchecked. The initial treatment consists of attempting to control the nausea and vomiting with medication. Also helpful has been the emphasis of heavier meals eaten before treatments and light meals after treatment. The choice of bland but attractively served foods seems to help. Careful attention should be paid to the patient's eating habits and fluid intake. If the symptoms persist uncontrolled, therapy may be interrupted and the patient maintained by intravenous feedings to replace lost electrolytes and nutrients. Interruption of therapy can greatly extend the patient's hospital stay and further interrupt normal activity. It is important that the nurse be cognizant of impending problems for the patient, guard against them, and report them early so that optimum health can be maintained and there will be a good prospect of returning more quickly to as normal a way of life as possible.

Skin reaction to radiation is still another area of concern to the nursing staff. The skin may often darken in the area of radiation and may become more tender and prone to breakdown, with subsequent infection and healing problems. Care should be taken not to use greasy or oily substances or powders on the affected skin, since they are hard to clean from the skin and often have metal substances in their makeup that can increase the concentration of radiation in the treatment area, compounding the existing problem. The treatment of choice consists of keeping the skin cleansed with mild soap and water and then drying it carefully. If an ointment is needed for comfort or lubrication, the use of Aquaphor or a similar water-soluble substance is preferred. In addition, the nurse should carefully guard against excessive or prolonged pressure to these areas. If the vulva is included in the radiation field, the tissue usually responds with marked erythema and edema. With the development of brisk erythema, the treatment is usually interrupted until the tissues return to normal. Careful thought and action should be taken by the nursing staff to prevent skin complications that can lead to infection and again to prolonged hospital confinement.

Bone marrow depression is another problem inherent in external therapy to the pelvis. The white blood cell count and platelet count are carefully monitored once or twice weekly. If the white blood cell count drops to 2000, the therapy is interrupted to allow the bone marrow to regenerate and thus prevent irreversible thrombocytopenia and agranulocytosis, which would leave the patient prey to problems of bleeding and systemic infection.

If symptoms reach a severity that is uncontrollable, the therapy may be discontinued and other treatment modalities considered. For some patients there may not be any additional therapy. The majority of patients, under close and careful supervision, tolerate external radiation therapy well and are treated over a span of 5 to 7 weeks, depending on the dosage required. The average tolerable dose we are giving for gynecologic malignancy is from 5000 to 6000 rads.

Alone or in combination with external radiation therapy, intracavitary radiation may be used in patients having a cancer of the cervix, uterus, or vagina. The average time spent with each treatment is 60 to 72 hours, with the patient on bedrest. An indwelling catheter is placed and the bowel evacuated to prevent increased radiation exposure to the bowel or bladder due to distention. The side effects are less severe than external radiation, but the possible complications include uterine perforation and irritation to the bladder or bowel due to poor placement in proximity to these structures. Placement films are taken with each application, and the equipment is checked frequently for proper positioning. The patient undergoes one to three treatments, usually spaced 2 weeks apart. Premature removal of the radium device is performed if the patient has an elevated temperature, severe abdominal pain, bloating, or severe diarrhea. The remaining hours of treatment can be given at a later date.

Treatment is discussed thoroughly with the patient so that she understands the possible complications and damage, as well as the extent of her involvement and hospital stay during her treatments. This information enables her to make more realistic plans with her family and friends in carrying through activities for which she is normally responsible and in changing her life patterns while she is undergoing therapy, as well as preparing her for possible impending problems so that she and the staff are aware of them before they become severe and impede her quicker recovery.

Surgery

Surgical procedures for use in gynecologic cancer may range from conization in carcinoma in situ lesions of the cervix, as mentioned earlier, to vaginal hysterectomy, total abdominal hysterectomy with bilateral salpingo-oophorectomy, or modified radical or radical hysterectomy, which adds a lymphadenectomy to the above procedure. Included under radical procedures are pelvic exenteration, either total, anterior, or posterior; total vaginectomy; and vulvectomy with pelvic lymphadenectomy. The exenteration involves interruption of the function of either the bladder or bowel, or both, with the formation of an ileal conduit and/or colostomy. It also includes a total or an approximately total vaginectomy, which will cause interruption of vaginal sexual intercourse for the patient. Much counseling and teaching is necessary for those patients, not only in regard to the changes they face in physiologic functioning and how to take care of themselves, but also in regard to their continued relationships to significant others. These patients need the security of being loved and need help in recognizing themselves as still functioning and worthwhile human beings. Plans and counseling for this kind of help from the health care team must begin before surgery. Loved ones should be included in these plans at the earliest possible point, and nurses are in a good position to be responsible for instigating this kind of help. If planning is begun after surgery, a lot of time and patient strength can be lost or wasted.

The vulvectomy, which includes removal of the vulva and lymph nodes and shortening of the vagina and urethra, carries with it a high rate of morbidity due to wound breakdown of a very large wound, which usually lengthens the patient's hospital stay. Lymphedema of the lower extremities may also cause difficulty in returning to many occupations. Once the wound is healed, normal activity, including sexual relation, is encouraged for the patient. The problems of changes in self-image and life-style that are found in exenteration must also be considered for the vulvectomy patient. Many patients return to full activity, and there have been reported cases of young women who have become mothers, with a normal delivery, after vulvectomy. For a quick return to normalcy, help should be available at the earliest possible point, again by means counseling and giving information in a caring relationship before surgery.

In addition to complications previously mentioned for radiation therapy and surgery are those found to arise from a combination of the two modalities. If a patient has had surgery before radiation therapy, proctitis as well as other gastrointestinal symptoms may be found to be more severe. It is believed that the reason lies in the formation of adhesions postoperatively, causing the bowel to be held in place so that certain loops receive heavy irradiation. Severe damage and obstruction eventually follow if symptoms are not observed and treated carefully. Patients are often older and may be obese. If radiation, with its tissue changes, precedes surgery, the most prevalent complication can be poor wound healing. Retention sutures are often used to prevent evisceration in the face of possible dehiscence. It is imperative that daily scrupulous monitoring and cleansing of the wound be done to prevent infection and wound breakdown, which will result in increased morbidity and lengthening of the hospital stay.

At all times the health care team must be aware of the possible outcomes of treatment for cure and what impact those outcomes will have on the patient's self-respect and self-image, as well as the demands that will be made for a change in life-style. Of course, the patient and health care team will be pleased with the probability of eradicating the cancer, but after, depending on the extent of treatment, there is much work to be done to build a new life that is happy and rewarding rather than accepting an existence that may be demeaning to the patient. Nurses should be aware of impending or possible problems and plan early with the patient, before treatment begins, for the help that will be necessary during treatment and after its completion.

HOW THE PATIENT'S DISEASE IS CONTROLLED

For many persons a cure for their cancer is simply not available. At this point the health care team looks at ways in which the growth of the cancer might be retarded or controlled and in which treatment side effects and discomfort may be held to a minimum. Not so long ago a prevalent concern of the health team was to maintain "life" at all cost, even when continued existence was abhorrent to the individual patient. Today many health care workers are concerned with the maintenance of a quality of life rather than a quantity of life. Certainly for all of us, but particularly for patients who are receiving palliative treatment, each day should have its own importance, and thought should be given not only to the possible extension of time but to guarding against "wasting" that time.

All three modalities of treatment—radiation therapy, chemotherapy, and surgery—are used in palliation of incurable gynecologic cancers. Many times they are used in combination. For instance, in extensive involvement in ovarian carcinoma, surgery is performed to debulk the greater mass of the tumor. After the wound has healed the patient is then treated with radiation therapy and chemotherapy, many times with a good response that not only has made the patient more comfortable but has on occasion increased her life span by several years with minimal symptoms. For many of the cancers in gynecology, when they are inoperable and radiation therapy either has already been used or cannot be used, chemotherapy has been the treatment of choice to help retard the cancer's growth. For carcinoma of the vulva, a simple vulvectomy may be performed to remove a fungating mass, or when the mass is too extensive and there is distance matastasis, radiation may be used to shrink and dry the mass so that comfort is provided for the patient. Relief may be obtained from obstruction of the bowel due to pressure from the tumor mass. The smaller the tumor mass left behind, the more responsive the tumor will be to either radiation therapy or chemotherapy, or both.

Many physicians make an attempt to limit the amount of time the patient has to spend being treated for palliation so that the patient may return to a more normal way of life as quickly as possible. Nurses can plan ahead for the patient's needs when she returns home, so that the transition from hospital to home is smooth, with resources for meeting both physical and emotional needs readily available. The nurse must spend time planning, with the patient, what needs the patient will have and what kinds of help are available to her. Consultation with the social service department on available community assistance, job placement, social activities, financial assistance, and family support systems, to name a few areas in which help may be needed, is important in planning with the patient for a stable and secure environment. Referrals to the visiting nurse association in regard to the patient's health care needs can provide for support and assistance in the home setting. Involvement of the clergy, if the patient receives support from this avenue, can be instituted by the nurse. Provision should be made for necessary supplies so that the patient need not worry about obtaining them. Occasionally the patient may require such care that, rather than returning home, she must be placed in a nursing home. Plans in all instances should have patient input, when possible, to give her as much independence of action as is feasible in her situation.

SUMMARY

All patients coming to the health care team for treatment for cure or palliation of their cancer are first of all human beings who have a right to exert as much control over their situation as possible. No patient should undergo treatment or care before plans are made to rehabilitate and maintain her at the highest possible level of both physical and psychologic wholeness. In caring for the patient with cancer, clinicians must be cognizant of the effects of treatment or lack of treatment and the resulting changes in the patient's life pattern. With these changes in mind, it is then necessary to start planning with the patient not only for her care but for her return to "hope" and "life."

Part of rehabilitation involves fully informing the patient so that she can make realistic decisions on her own behalf, based on what she wants from that future and from the people that can help her. A consistent approach is necessary in building a trusting relationship that can last throughout treatment and subsequent care. Even with added information and trust, the patient may still desire that no treatment be undertaken. This can often be seen in the patient with more extensive disease. Once that decision is made, the patient should never be abandoned in favor of those who seek treatment, nor should she be cut off from a future attempt at palliation. She needs support through the decision-making process, and just as the health care team members work through treatment complications with their patients, so should they be available to work through with patients the complications of extended and untreated disease. The patient should feel and know that the health team will be available for whatever assistance is needed, whenever she seeks that assistance.

It is up to the nurse to help the patient set realistic goals for a future with some quality and purpose, no matter how long that future may be. Plans need to be made for continued support and feedback for the patient, and the nurse can be the instigator for bringing together all those persons, abilities, strengths, and desires that can lead to a better way of life. First, the nurse must have a reverence for life that does not waste it and a respect for the individual as an independent and self-directed being. Furthermore, the nurse must know the available resources for assistance and how best to use them to return the patient to her optimum state of functioning and being.

REFERENCES

1. Barckley, V.: The crisis in cancer, American Journal of Nursing **67**:278-280, Feb., 1967.
2. George, M, and McGrath, M. S.: Long-term care of the patient with cancer, Nursing Clinics of North America **8**: Dec., 1973.
3. Gynecologic Cancer, ACOG Technical Bulletin, No. 24, Aug., 1973, pp. 1-7.
4. Knapp, R. C., and Valentina, D. D.: Gynecologic surgery: it's threat to sexuality, Consultant **12**:55-56, Aug., 1972.

19 Child with cancer

facilitating the return to school*

ELISE T. WEAR
PATRICIA BLESSING

On a fall day in 1973 we received a telephone call from the local schoolteacher of one of our patients. Tommy was a recently hospitalized 7-year-old by who had acute lymphocytic leukemia. The local teacher said in a distraught voice, "Why didn't you prepare me for Tommy's return to school? He can hardly walk! He looks so different, so bloated, but Tom says he feels much better! His mother tells me that she wants him in school. What am I supposed to do with him? How am I going to explain this to the other children?"

This phone conversation led us to wonder whether other teachers of our patients had similar problems. We also thought that the distress shown by this teacher probably created difficulties for Tommy.

For several years as professionals representing different disciplines, we had worked closely together in caring for children with cancer. We shared a belief that school, with its opportunity for learning and social interaction, was essential for promoting growth and development of all children, including those with cancer. The nursing care of the hospitalized child provided uninterrupted time for school each weekday if the child felt well enough for this experience. After discharge from the hospital, the child was encouraged to reenter his local school as soon as he was physically able. We believed that a satisfying school experience added significantly to the quality of life for a child affected with a malignant condition.

As we conferred about the problem that Tommy's teacher had shared, we hypothesized the following:

1. Local schoolteachers had had little or no experience and instruction in teaching children who have cancer.

2. The return of an affected child to school creates stress for the teacher, child, parents, and classmates.

3. Having a child with cancer in school can be a rewarding experience for all.

4. Various interventions by hospital staff with the child, the parents, and the

_____

*Research supported in part by a grant from the National Cancer Institute to the Wisconsin Clinical Cancer Center, No. P02-CA-14520.

local school personnel would reduce the stress factors and assist the child with cancer and the school personnel to meet their needs.

The purpose of this chapter is to discuss our experiences with developing interventions that promote coping strategies in these children and their local school personnel when the children reenter their home school.

VALIDATING OUR HYPOTHESES

Before helpful interventions could be developed, we decided that the aforementioned hypotheses needed to be validated. We therefore undertook a four-pronged study consisting of the following:

1. A review of the literature
2. A review of hospital practices to determine what interventions were being used and whether they were helpful
3. An assessment of our patients' attendance and performance at school
4. A polling of local schoolteachers to learn their perceptions and needs

We include the results of this study to provide a background for the interventions that were developed and, hopefully, to allow the reader to share our excitement as changes occurred that improved the school experience of our patients.

In searching the literature we found limited sources concerning the child with cancer returning to school. Robbins and Kacen,[3] Cyphert,[1] and Kaplan and colleagues[2] agreed that schooling for these children is important and challenging for the patient, the parents, and the school personnel. No literature gave specific suggestions about ways to facilitate a child's reentry into a class.

Robbins and Kacen,[3] writing in *Today's Education,* verified the hypothesis that little was taught in education courses relating to chronic illnesses. They stated that "the emphasis is solely on learning disabilities, not physical disabilities." Cyphert[1] supports this contention in his article "Back to School for the Child with Cancer," when he suggests that "many young teachers have never seen death intimately, and their training has not prepared them to handle it." He also states, "Elementary and secondary school educators are not being prepared by schools of education to handle the problems of chronically or terminally ill children."

The aforementioned authors substantiate the stress factors involved when a child with a malignancy returns to school. Robbins and Kacen[3] note that the child, the parents, and the teacher are fearful and anxious. They discuss several psychologic reactions, principally denial, guilt, and anger, exhibited by the parents. Affected children, too, experience these reactions along with self-doubt, all of which influence their behavior and performance in school. Cyphert[1] describes teachers' feelings well when he says, "We don't know what to say to him, so we say little; we fear that we might get asked an uncomfortable question so we don't permit the opportunity for questions; we overempathize because we identify the child with cancer with our own loved ones."

Kaplan and associates[2] acknowledge that the child's ability to cope with a serious illness is largely dependent on the behavior of adults in the immediate environment. These authors state that "becoming aware of protective responses" may be the first step in controlling adult anxiety.

None of the literature addressed the subject of the potential rewards of having a child with cancer in school.

Our review of hospital practices showed that nurses and hospital teachers were involved in helping the child with the school experience. At that time, three public-school teachers were assigned to teach at our children's hospital. These teachers helped all hospitalized school-age children to proceed with their learning and maintain their class level. During a child's hospitalization, the hospital teacher phoned each patient's local teacher or guidance counselor. The child's school performance was discussed and the hospital lessons were coordinated with those of the home class. At discharge, the hospital teacher sent the local school a report of the patient's academic progress. In this report the hospital teacher discussed any concerns and anxieties that the child had about returning to school.

As part of the planning for discharge from the hospital, nurses talked with the child and the parents about returning to school. This discussion included such topics as when the child would medically be able to reenter school, how the child planned to handle classmates' questions, and a suggestion that the parents talk with the school about the child's condition.

The children and parents appeared to appreciate this anticipatory guidance. Often the children were creative in their responses. One 12-year-old girl said, "I'm going to tell my best friend all about my illness and tell her to tell everyone else so I won't have to answer questions." A 9-year-old boy said, "I want you to tell my teacher that I've lost my hair again, and she should tell the kids and tell them I don't want to answer any questions!"

The majority of children and parents stated that they felt confident in handling the reentry to the local school. As professionals, we shared their confidence. It seemed that nurturing independence on the part of parents and children would be therapeutic and a valid medical/educational goal. Furthermore, the hematology-oncology team of health professionals included the patient and family in decision making. The child and parents were encouraged to become as knowledgeable as they wished about the child's illness and care, and information about the patient's condition was freely shared. Thus, from the point of view of the hospital staff, many of the children and their parents became medically sophisticated. It was thought that with the above-mentioned anticipatory guidance, the patient would be able to return to the local school comfortably.

However, it became apparent that such a pleasant outcome was rarely achieved. When the children came to clinic, outpatient nurses inquired about their performance and attendance at school, and the children or their parents reported school problems, even when the child's disease was under control. Some children were functioning below their known level of academic ability, and others attended irregularly because they were teased or because the parents thought that teachers did not set reasonable expectations. A few parents said that because they were unable to deal with the school, they chose not to send their child to school.

While data were being gathered, we sought information about local teachers' feelings, needs, and practices when our patients reentered their classes. The hospital teacher conferred with some teachers in schools throughout our midwestern state. These teachers agreed that they had little or no experience in dealing with children who have a malignant condition, and they shared their anxiety about teaching such a child. Some seemed to believe that coping with physical disabilities was not their responsibility; the child's academic performance was their concern. They said that they assumed the school nurse would handle "the rest."

Concurrently with this verbal input, a questionnaire was sent to a small sampling of community-based teachers of children who had been hospitalized on the hematology-oncology service within the first 8 months of 1974.

The questionnaire was designed to elicit such information as how the teacher learned of the child's diagnosis; whether the school nurse was involved; how the affected child adjusted to school; whether the children in the class were informed of their classmate's problem and, if so, by whom; whether the teacher discussed the child's illness with the class; how the class reacted to the affected child and his illness; and whether the teacher desired information (help) from the hospital staff and, if so, what kind?

All the questionnaires were returned. The replies confirmed the need to help the children and their local school personnel. The teachers who responded taught in kindergarten through grade 4. Over half had not previously had a child with an ongoing illness in their class. One school nurse was involved. Many children learned of their classmate's illness from their parents or through community gossip. The consensus was that most children were told that the disease was fatal and that the child would die soon. A few teachers reported that they attempted to discuss hospitals, serious illness, and treatments that cause alterations in physical appearance.

Some teachers stated that the affected child returned to school activities comfortably, and that classmates welcomed the child and tried to be helpful. Other teachers were vehement about how difficult the adjustment was for all concerned. For instance, several teachers wrote that the returning child seemed to believe that rules were for others to obey. For example: "He hit other children but felt he shouldn't be hit"; "he refused to complete assignments."

Some teachers said that the child's appearance caused concern. They reported that teasing occurred on the playground or in the halls about the affected child's baldness, changes in weight, or difficulty in running.

All respondents to the questionnaire stated that they needed written explanations by health professionals about the child's illness and treatment. Unanimously, they said that the information should be given by hospital personnel rather than parents, since the former "could be more objective." The teachers asked how the illness and treatment would influence the child's school performance, stamina, and attitude in the classroom.

DEVELOPING INTERVENTIONS

After studying this material, we concluded that our hypotheses were valid, with the possible exception of the statement that "having a child with cancer in school can be a rewarding experience for all." We had no data to substantiate this hypothesis other than our own beliefs. For us, working with these children is rewarding. We find that, with skillful assistance, they usually develop an amazing ability to cope with their own tragic situations. Our rewards come from seeing these children, with our help, adapt in a courageous manner. Therefore the major determinant appears to be possessing the knowledge and skills to help the child develop coping strategies. Germane to this chapter is the knowledge of how to facilitate a patient's reentry to his local school. The data we had obtained directed the development of several interventions to be used by nurses and schoolteachers.

First, the data suggested that nurses could be more comprehensive in their patient/parent guidance about the child's return to the local school. Thus, after a brain-storming session with staff nurses, the following list of topics was developed to be discussed with the child and parents near the time of discharge from the hospital:

1. When the child would medically be able to reenter school
2. Any restrictions on the child's activity or diet that should be shared with the school, and how the child and parents thought this information could best be given to the school
3. What the child and parents thought the school should know about the child's illness and treatment
4. Difficulties the child or parents anticipate in the return to school, and ways that nursing personnel can be of help
5. How to help the child think through what to say in response to questions about the hospitalization, illness, or such changes in appearance as hair loss, weight gain or loss, and scars
6. An offer to talk with the local teacher about any concerns the child or parents have if desired
7. A suggestion that parents discuss with the local school nurse the child's condition, plans for ongoing care and medications, and their concerns about the child's school experience

For the past several months staff nurses have included this procedure in their nursing care. They report a gratifying response by the patients and their parents. The staff nurses say that they are enthusiastic about this intervention because they believe it provides better nursing care.

Second, it seemed that a method for establishing an ongoing relationship with local schools was needed. We decided that telephone conferences between the hospital staff and the local school personnel might serve this purpose. Therefore, a nurse and/or a hospital teacher talks with the patient and the parents about our desire to help the child reenter the local school and to ask their permission to contact that school. The majority of children and parents support this practice enthusiastically.

If permission is obtained while the child is hospitalized, at least one telephone conference is held between the hospital nurse/teacher team and the local school personnel—teacher, principal, school nurse, and/or guidance counselor. During this conference the nurse usually is asked to review the nature of the child's dis-

---

School _____

City _____

    Your student, _____, is currently under the care of the Hematology-Oncology Department at University Children's Hospital. In an effort to provide a smooth reentry into your classroom and in response to data gathered from teachers, we are enclosing information concerning this child's illness. This is being done with the permission of the child's parents. However, we assume that you will regard it as a confidential report.

    It has been established that the child with a malignant disease who is well enough to be in school can continue to learn and enjoy learning. It is felt that such children should be treated as much like normal children as possible, since school is a major part of a normal child's life. Normalcy in life-style is most important to the sick child's needs. Being in school and engaged in learning has been very helpful in such children's adjustments. It is believed that the quality of school life is vital to mental health, which significantly affects physical health.

    We have found that there is no definitive formula for teaching these children. The nature and degree of the disease are significant, and factors that affect learning may consequently change. A careful study and evaluation of such children's abilities, attitudes, and learning patterns before the illness is helpful in teaching the child when he returns. While the child is hospitalized, the hematology-oncology team encourages the child and parents to play an active part in decision making. It has been found that the most successful reentries of children into their classrooms occur when the child, the parents, and the teachers can continue to function as a team to establish valid expectations for the child.

    Experience tells us that the child's classmates need to be prepared for the sick child's return. It is hoped that the enclosed explanation of the illness can be interpreted to the group by the teacher on the appropriate level of understanding. It is also important for other faculty members and school personnel to be prepared for the child's return.

    It is believed that if this child is to have a successful return to school, good communication and cooperation between health personnel and educators are essential. We realize that oftentimes school personnel are not experienced in handling cases of children with serious illnesses. Therefore, if you have any questions, please feel free to telephone one of the persons listed below. We would appreciate the completion of the enclosed evaluation sheet so that we can continue in our attempt to help children and teachers.

ease, the treatment, and the prognosis. The hospital teacher discusses the child's academic progress. We try to prepare the local school personnel for any changes in the child's appearance and to establish a relationship that will be helpful to all by sharing concerns and questions. We encourage the school to call us at any time, emphasizing that we appreciate suggestions about how we can be more helpful.

The telephone conferences have been exciting. Usually the local school personnel sound at ease and eager for information. We believe that many beneficial relationships have begun through this intervention. However, since this practice has been in use for only 6 months, the definitive results are not known.

Third, the data clearly indicate that local schools want written information about the child. We concluded that three forms of written communication would be assistive. One such communication is the letter shown on p. 227 to the child's schoolteacher from the hospital teacher.

Although this letter is signed by the hospital teacher, the names and telephone numbers of all the schoolteachers and all the members of the hematology-oncology team are listed.

Another form explains the child's illness, whether it is leukemia or a malignant tumor, in language that can be understood by lay persons. The fact that these diseases are noncommunicable and nonhereditary is stressed. The treatment is noted in a generalized manner, and the common side effects are listed and explained. In the hope of portraying an accurate picture of these diseases and their treatment, the following statement is given: "The aim of treatment is to return the child to normal or near normal function, but from time to time the child may experience some side effects that will prohibit full function. The outlook for children with this disease with modern therapy is much better than it was in the past. When cure is not possible, attempts are made to keep the illness under control for varying periods of time."

The last form of written communication is a checklist, as shown on opposite page. We hoped that this style of material would be used easily by a busy classroom teacher.

This checklist is completed quickly by nursing and educational personnel at the time of a patient's discharge. Often the child and his parents add their comments to be shared with the local teacher.

The majority of children and their parents have expressed appreciation for these interventions. Only one family refused this kind of assistance, saying that they would handle the situation themselves. Some parents have chosen to read the written material carefully before giving their consent. Other parents have preferred that the nurse or teacher summarize it verbally. Some parents did not want to know the content of the forms. They said, "I trust you. If you think this is best for my child, go ahead and send it." Usually the children glanced at the pages briefly and gave their permission by saying "okay."

In addition to the three forms of written information, an evaluation sheet and a self-addressed stamped envelope are sent to the local school. In this evaluation

---

Information about _____

At time of discharge _____

Description	Yes	No	Comments
Change in appearance			
Hair loss			_____
Weight change			_____
Bruises present			_____
Change in muscular control			
Diminished fine motor			_____
Diminished gross motor			_____
Restrictions in physical education classes			_____
Restrictions in playground activities			_____
Dietary restrictions			_____
Medication to be taken during school			_____

This checklist applies to the present and will change in varying lengths of time. Again, we suggest that you consult the child and the parents if you have any questions.

---

we ask the local teacher to assess the telephone conference and the written forms, to discuss how the child behaved and performed on reentry into school, to comment on the classmates' reactions to the returning child, and to state whether the child and the parents are involved in making decisions about the child's school experience.

At the time of writing this chapter, few of these evaluation forms have been returned. However, those which we have received and verbal reports from schools have been encouraging and reinforcing.

To illustrate the implementation of these interventions, we include the story of Darla, a 13-year-old girl with Hodgkin's disease. Darla was hospitalized for 8 weeks, during which time a diagnosis was established, radiotherapy was given, and anti-tumor medications were started. By the time she left the hospital she had lost her hair, but she had an attractive wig that she wore except when she was asleep.

While she was hospitalized, Darla, her nurse, and her mother talked together about her life with Hodgkin's disease and its treatment. Particularly, Darla discussed how she would handle any questioning or teasing by classmates. She decided to be open and truthful about what had happened to her. However, she was concerned about her return to school because it was necessary for her to attend a new school in a new city. She had been in this school only a few weeks before she entered the hospital, and she did not think that she had friends in the school.

After obtaining permission from Darla and her mother, the nurse and the hospital-school teacher conferred by telephone with her eighth-grade homeroom teacher and the school nurse. When Darla's concerns were discussed, the local school personnel seemed understanding and said that they were eager for Darla to return. Since they asked for written information, we sent to them the three forms that we had developed.

As Darla was leaving the hospital she reiterated that she felt well prepared for reentry into her community and school. However, when she went to school, she found that her new classmates teased her until she could not bear it. She said, "I was ready for some teasing, but they called me 'baldy' so often and tried to snatch my wig off."

When Darla refused to go to school, the school nurse called us for suggestions. After conferring on the telephone, we concluded that a discussion of Darla's disease and its treatment might help her and her classmates. Darla, her teacher, and her school nurse planned and conducted a class on Hodgkin's disease as part of the science curriculum. Darla proudly relates how the students asked her questions and how she answered them. The teasing stopped, and now Darla says that she enjoys school. Her teachers report that she is progressing well, and she attends regularly.

Certainly, Darla and her school coped with the situation in a creative manner. We were gratified to hear that the school personnel thought our verbal and written information was essential in helping them to assist Darla. Hopefully, after this experience, having Darla in that school will be rewarding for all concerned.

In summary, we want to emphasize that it is too early to thoroughly evaluate the effectiveness of the aforementioned interventions. We anticipate that changes will be made as we learn from our patients, their parents, and their schools. However, we would like to encourage the reader to use any of the described interventions found helpful. We are convinced that they promote the development of coping strategies in children with cancer and in their local school personnel.

REFERENCES

1. Cyphert, F. R.: Back to school for the child with cancer, Proceedings of the American Cancer Society's National Conference on Human Values and Cancer, p. 134, June 22-24, 1972.
2. Kaplan, D. M., Smith, A., and Grobstein, R.: School management of the seriously ill child, The Journal of School Health **44:** 251, May, 1974.
3. Robbins, L. R., and Kacen, N. M.: How should the teacher view the chronically ill pupil? Todays Education, pp. 28-35, May, 1971.